All you ever wanted to know about
VITAMINS

by Dr Leonard Mervyn
BSc, PhD

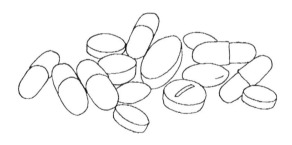

Published by
Amberwood Publishing Ltd
Guildford, England

PLANTLIFE

The Natural History Museum, Cromwell Road, London SW7 5BD

Registered Charity No. 328576

Amberwood Publishing supports the Plantlife Charity,
Britain's only charity exclusively dedicated to saving wild plants.

ISBN 1-899308-22-9

Cover production by Howland Northover

Printed in Great Britain

CONTENTS

Note to Reader

About the Author

Dr. Leonard Mervyn is a Clinical Biochemist, experienced in pharmaceutical research and with a special interest in Vitamins and Minerals. He was the first to discover Coenzyme Q10 in man and identified the active form of vitamin B12, methylcobalamin, in human blood. He has written many books and scientific papers and has been honoured both by a Cressy Morrison Award from the New York Academy of Sciences and by an Italseber Gold Medal from the University of Pavia. Dr. Mervyn was an external examiner for Oxford University and visiting lecturer at the University of Kingston and is currently the Technical Director of a major healthcare company.

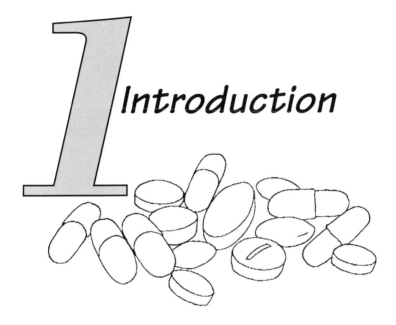

1 Introduction

The term vitamin is attributed to the Polish chemist Casimir Funk who coined it from "vita" (meaning life), and "amine" (a class of chemical substances to which vitamins were assigned, albeit incorrectly). Funk merely put a name to a concept of micronutrients, usually present in food, that are essential to maintain health in animals and man. This idea was originally suggested by the British biochemist, Sir Frederick Gowland Hopkins.

Strictly speaking, a true vitamin should satisfy certain criteria before being acceptable as such, and these are:

1. They are needed only in small amounts.
2. Adequate amounts should be supplied in the diet.
3. When they are deficient the individual shows distinct clinical symptoms and disease.
4. That disease and these symptoms are cured only by treatment with that specific vitamin.

As we shall see, these are only generalizations since there are exceptions to every criterion. For example, certain fats and amino acids (from proteins) are essential for health and can only be obtained from the diet, but the relatively large quantities needed puts them outside the first criterion, although they satisfy the other three. Some vitamins are made within the body, either in the tissues themselves or by bacteria that inhabit the intestine, but it is debatable whether sufficient for the body's needs can be met in this way. A deficiency of a single vitamin of the vitamin B complex is rare so symptoms may be related to lack of more than one. Similarly, treatment to overcome these symptoms may require multi-vitamin therapy, although in specific cases only one vitamin need be given.

In the early days of vitamin research, vitamins were conveniently put into one of two categories, namely, fat-soluble and water-soluble. Although this separated them on the basis of their physical property, later studies indicated the two types were also different in their functions within the body. We shall see later what these are, but let us first look at the vitamins we know exist.

The fat-soluble vitamins are designated A, D, E and K. There is also beta-carotene known as a provitamin because the body can convert it to vitamin A. Although this is an important source of the vitamin in vegetarians and vegans because they are not eating pre-formed vitamin A found only in foods of animal, fish and poultry origins, beta–carotene has important functions in its own right. These include its protective function in the body as an antioxidant, as are vitamins C and E. Certain *polyunsaturated fatty acids* were once known as Vitamin F but this designation is falling into disuse to be replaced by the term *EFA* or *Essential Fatty Acids*. The required daily intake of EFA is measured in grams which rather puts them outside the province of true vitamins despite their being necessary for health.

The water-soluble vitamins consist of the members of the vitamin B complex and vitamin C. The vitamin B complex consists of eight, eleven or thirteen members, depending upon which authority you believe. For the purpose of this book we shall regard the true vitamin B complex as a mixture of *eight* different substances. The other possible members are still in contention but we shall consider their possible therapeutic uses later.

The eight true vitamins in the B complex are thiamine (vitamin B1), *riboflavine* (vitamin B2), *niacin* (vitamin B3), *pantothenic acid* (vitamin B5), *pyridoxine* (vitamin B6), *cobalamin* (vitamin B12), *folic acid and biotin*. The three members loosely associated with the complex are *choline, inositol* and *para-aminobenzoic acid (PABA)*. You will see that the trivial names are given first with the appropriate number in parentheses. This is because there is now an increasing tendency to characterise vitamins by name in the regulations laid down by various authorities so as to avoid past ambiguities in the numbering of the members of the vitamin B complex.

One reason why the first eight members of the vitamin B complex fall neatly into one category is because they all function in a similar manner. To explain this we must look at the fundamental principle of life itself.

All forms of life, ranging from the simple one-cell organisms, like yeasts or bacteria, to the highly complex human being, are based on a mass of biochemical reactions. Life itself depends upon these chemical changes which regulate the way we digest food and break it down into simpler components; the way these nutrients are turned into energy; the way this energy translates into the movement of life; the way the biochemicals in food enable the brain and nervous system to function; the way essential nutrients are built up into new blood, flesh and other tissues. These biochemical reactions actually determine the processes upon which life is sustained. However, they cannot occur at a rate to sustain life without a catalyst to speed up these processes.

Substances that produce chemical change in the body, and indeed in any living thing, are known as *enzymes*. They are sometimes referred to as *organic catalysts* or *accelerators*, but whatever the name, the function is the same, to quicken life's processes. Enzymes are all specific types of *proteins* and we rely upon the body to produce its own supply of them. Unfortunately, most of these enzymes cannot function alone as they require some other factors to help them perform their roles. These factors are known as *coenzymes*, and these in turn are *vitamins*, usually those of the vitamin B complex.

It is easy to see, therefore, how important vitamins are to the processes of life. Without vitamins, life-sustaining reactions slow down because the enzymes cannot function without their coenzymes. Symptoms of ill-health will follow and eventually death may result. Adequate intakes of the B vitamins are hence necessary on a regular basis to ensure body levels are maintained at a suitable level. Fortunately, enzymes and coenzymes (vitamins) are not destroyed when they are performing their life-giving functions and are used over and over again. However, some losses, due mainly to excretion of vitamins, are inevitable, so without a constant dietary intake a slow, insidious deficiency will result.

Although much is known about the functions of the vitamin B complex as coenzymes, the other vitamins appear to work in other ways. Vitamins C and E, for example, have important protective roles within the body; vitamin C in the fluid of the organs and vitamin E in the fatty tissues. Vitamin K has one unique function, that of ensuring the clotting capacity of the blood is maintained. Vitamin A supports a healthy skin, mucous (wet) membranes and eyes, as well as performing a unique role in the process of sight. Vitamin D is solely concerned with ensuring efficient absorption of calcium and phosphorus from the diet. In none of their functions do these vitamins appear to act as coenzymes but rather directly or indirectly as essential substances in their own right.

When we look at our minimum needs of these essential vitamins on a daily basis the surprising thing to emerge is the vast variation in their quantities required. At the two extremes are vitamin C at about 100 milligrams (one three-hundredth of an ounce), or one-tenth of one gram, and vitamin B12 at one microgram, or one millionth of one gram. The others fall somewhere in between. These differences may reflect the proportionate amounts present in the food and probably represent how man has aligned to his diet over the millions of years of evolution. What is highly significant is that the inability to absorb just one-millionth of one gram of vitamin B12 daily leads to just as grave consequences as does the lack of the other vitamins needed in much larger amounts. All are important for health – none can replace another.

A note on vitamin measurement
You may come across vitamins expressed as international units (i.u.) as well as or instead of weight (milligrams or micrograms). International units are a left-over from the days of vitamin research when the chemical structures of the micronutrients were unknown and scientists measured them in terms of biological activity, i.e. their effect upon some physiological function of an animal. Later as they were isolated and as their structures became known, vitamins could be measured in terms of their weight and international units became obsolete. Nevertheless, some have persisted and, today, vitamins A, D and E may be expressed in international units on labels. The relationships are as follows:

VITAMIN A 1 microgram = 3.33 i.u.
VITAMIN D 1 microgram = 40 i.u.
VITAMIN E 1 milligram = 1 i.u. dl-alpha tocopheryl acetate
VITAMIN E 1 milligram = 1.36 i.u. d-alpha tocopheryl acetate
VITAMIN E 1 milligram = 1.1 i.u. dl-alpha tocopherol
VITAMIN E 1 milligram = 1.49 i.u. d-alpha tocopherol
VITAMIN E 1 milligram = 0.89 i.u. dl-alpha tocopheryl succinate
VITAMIN E 1 milligram = 1.21 i.u. d-alpha tocopheryl succinate

Note
1 gram (g) = 1000 milligrams (mg)
1 milligram (mg) = 1000 micrograms (μg)
1 kilogram (kg) = 1000 grams (g)

In Europe it has been shown by market research that between 10 and 15% of the population take some sort of vitamin/mineral supplement on a regular basis. Yet in North America at least 40% of the US population already take vitamin/mineral supplements of which 53% are 'multi' and 41% are specific micro nutrient preparations. These are taken in the main as preventive measures against the serious diseases of later life but many are taken also to replenish vitamins and minerals lost to excess by various lifestyles. Although the perfect diet would provide 215mg vitamin C, 23mg vitamin E, 6mg beta-carotene, 350μg folic acid and 1000mg calcium with Recommended Dietary Allowances (RDA's) of all the other vitamins and minerals, such figures are achievable only through supplementation either by tablets or fortification of foods.

The limiting nutrients in the typical American and European diets are folic acid, vitamin B6, magnesium and zinc. Second limiting are calcium, iron and the carotenoid sources of vitamin A. Economists have estimated that improved intakes of certain micro nutrients, in particular the antioxidants vitamin C, vitamin E and beta-carotene, would decrease healthcare costs by 25% for cardiovascular disease; by 16-30% for a variety of major cancers and by 50% for eye cataract conditions. These translate into billions of dollars of healthcare cost savings per annum. Adequate intakes of the necessary micro nutrients could be achieved by full restoration of the nutrient losses attributable to the refinement of wheat, corn and rice flour or by adding the appropriate vitamins and minerals to the refined foods. In addition, the needs for antioxidant nutrients which are far and above the dietary provision can only be achieved by tablet or capsule supplementation.

Supplemental use of vitamins to prevent disease is becoming more and more apparent . The efficacy of such use, or even the trend for intakes above that which can be supplied by means of diet alone, has been the source of considerable controversy in the medical and scientific fields. Recently published data has given strong support to several of the claims for major benefits of disease prevention, including that of cancer, cardiovascular disease, carpal tunnel syndrome and neural tube defects, to name just a few. The purported benefits for supplemental vitamin usage are discussed as well as how vitamins can complement medical therapy of these diseases.

Recent discoveries from the field of research include:

(i) How you may diagnose mild deficiencies of vitamins when induced by bad diets or one's own lifestyle.

(ii) How the RDAs are designed for levels of vitamin intake which can be achieved by means of diet, not for those wishing to prevent chronic diseases by means of vitamin supplementation.

(iii) Supplemental intakes of the antioxidant vitamins (C, E and beta-carotene) have been shown to reduce the risk of specific types of cancers and cardiovascular diseases.

(iv) Supplemental vitamin B6 may prevent the onset of carpal tunnel syndrome.

(v) Supplemental nicotinic acid, but not niacinamide, is effective in lowering blood cholesterol levels, especially that of low-density lipoprotein cholesterol.

(vi) Supplemental folic acid to women of childbearing age can reduce the risk of neural tube defects but poses the real risk of masking pernicious anaemia in the elderly.

One of the most bewildering aspects of vitamin and mineral supplementation to the average person is the vast range of potencies of these nutrients on display in any health food store and in some pharmacies. These products can be classed within three different levels of potency, each of which has a logical reason for taking it and so simplifying the process of selection.

The first of these can be described as products containing a comparatively low potency of ingredients and hence known as the Insurance level. These are usually present in at least 100% of the Recommended Daily Allowance but may rise to 200 or 300%. They are simply meant to top up any mild deficiency of nutrients due to inadequate diets of one sort or another. The intake is usually one capsule or tablet daily and this will ensure an adequate amount of ingredients for any individual without reference to those micro nutrients taken in the diet. These products are no substitute for a good diet but at least will guarantee there is no vitamin or mineral deficiency.

The second level of supplementation is what I call the 'Lifestyle' level and the potencies of the ingredients are usually between 400 and 500% of the RDA but may reach 1000% in some cases. The level is taken by those whose lifestyles require more vitamins than can be met even by a good diet. Such individuals may lead very stressful lives, can be tobacco smokers and/or drinkers of alcohol, are undergoing medical therapy on prescribed drugs (or simply taking the contraceptive pill) or are athletically minded with high physical activity. These are all lifestyle factors which can demand increased turnover of vitamins that cannot be met from the food.

The third level of supplementation is what I call the Therapeutic level. These are vitamins that are taken at high, though absolutely safe, intakes because they are acting as therapeutic drugs rather than vitamins. This aspect of supplementation is becoming more popular as research groups continue to report how vitamins can often complement conventional medicinal drug therapy in treating certain diseases.

I must add also that in the UK at least, every vitamin supplement on sale to the general public can be considered safe, even on long term usage, as long as it is taken in accordance with the instructions on the pack.

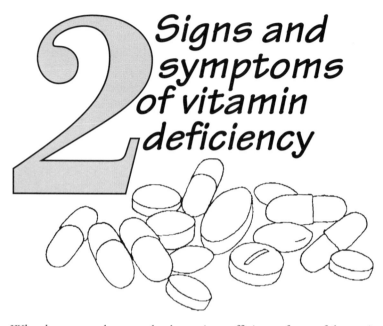

2 Signs and symptoms of vitamin deficiency

What happens when we don't receive sufficient of any of these vitamins? To answer this question we need to look at the difference between what is termed a gross deficiency, where the consequences may be life-threatening, and milder deficiencies where the consequences may be a feeling of 'under-the-weather' or, to steal another phrase, 'one degree under'. It is important to realise that the symptoms associated with a gross lack of vitamins may present themselves in a milder form with a less serious deficiency. Hence treatment is similar, namely replacement of the vitamin in short supply. We shall consider later how mild deficiencies may manifest themselves, but let us look at the gross deficiency disease.

We are very fortunate in the West that the diseases associated with serious deficiencies of various vitamins rarely present themselves, but they do exist in the world as a whole. Many thousands of people, particularly children, still go blind in Africa, Asia and South America because of vitamin A deficiency. Rickets, a disease specifically associated with lack of vitamin D, has reappeared in Britain amongst the Asian immigrant population. New-born babies, particularly premature ones, are increasingly being given small intramuscular injections of vitamins E and

K, to control the effects of excess oxygen and to prevent haemorrhage respectively – problems that may manifest themselves in the first few days of life. Vitamin B12 deficiency, usually due to an inability to absorb the vitamin, is still a world-wide problem. The end-result is pernicious anaemia, a killing form of anaemia, that is insidious in its onset.

Scurvy, once the scourge of sailors on long voyages, prevalent until less than 100 years ago, still reappears in early spring in elderly people in the northern hemispheres, and is due entirely to low intakes of vitamin C. Beriberi, induced by lack of thiamine (vitamin B1) is still the cause of death of many in the Third World although, mercifully, it is almost unknown in the West. Pellagra is a fatal disease that killed many thousands of Americans in the Southern states of the USA as recently as the 1920's. It was this tragedy that stimulated the American authorities to seek a reason for its prevalence. The culmination of their research was the demonstration that its prevention and cure was easily manifested by a substance called nicotinic acid – a chemical that had been known for more than 50 years at that time. Despite our knowledge on the relationship between pellagra and nicotinic acid, the disease still kills many thousands worldwide each year. In the UK, folic acid deficiency still represents a potential hazard in pregnancy, and recent research suggests a possible relationship between low maternal levels of the vitamin and the incidence of spina bifida in babies. The Department of Health now recommends increased intakes of folic acid by all women who are pregnant or contemplating pregnancy.

We need not feel complacent about not experiencing vitamin deficiency in the West, despite the fact that diseases due to gross deficiency are relatively rare. What is of more concern are those minor complaints that could be associated with a mild lack of certain vitamins. We shall consider these now but, before we do so, it is important to point out there is a growing belief amongst nutritionists, biochemists and some medical doctors that vitamin intake, and hence need, falls into two categories. In the first, low intake, there is just sufficient to prevent the signs and symptoms of gross vitamin deficiency from appearing. In the second, higher intake, there are sufficient vitamins to maintain optimum health. What most of us are getting is a vitamin intake somewhere in between these two levels. There are dietary means and perhaps supplementary treatment with vitamins to ensure that our intakes are at those required for optimum health. At the same time, we should not lose sight of the individual requirements of individuals in respect of their vitamin needs. Careful selection of supplementary vitamins may be required to satisfy particular demands by some people.

Symptoms possibly associated with vitamin deficiency

Mild abnormalities that may be associated with less serious deficiencies of vitamins are now being recognised in certain sectors of the population. Discrete areas of the body provide useful information to the individual so that with proper interpretation a clue to dietary deficiencies due to poor nutrition is given. At the same time, a superficial knowledge of what various vitamins do can indicate an associated possible deficiency if that particular function is affected. For example, the three B vitamins – thiamine, riboflavin and nicotinamide (or niacin) – are all concerned with the conversion of food to energy. Lack of energy may be due to mild deficiencies of these vitamins. Pyridoxine is the anti-depressant vitamin so any mild depressive state may respond to this vitamin. Pantothenic acid and biotin appear to have anti-stress functions so their intake should be increased in any stressful situation. Both vitamin B12 and folic acid are concerned with production of blood cells so they are useful factors in treating certain types of anaemia, themselves often a cause of tiredness and lack of energy. These are all symptoms that an individual can detect themselves, although professional help is essential to determine whether an anaemia is due to lack of vitamin B12 or of folic acid.

The more obvious areas affected by vitamin deficiencies are the skin, the mouth and the eyes but some symptoms of the gastro-intestinal tract and the nerves are also obvious to the individual affected. Many of these afflictions will respond to self-help in terms of improved diet or vitamin supplementation. Changes in the blood, the blood vessels, the heart, the bones, the brain and the reproductive systems that are associated with vitamin deficiency may require professional diagnosis. However, once diagnosis has been made, the individual can still confidently complement other treatments with improved diet and supplementary therapy as in heart disease, for example, where vitamin E, lecithin and fish oils will act in conjunction with conventional medical treatment.

The Skin

Animal studies have provided much of our knowledge on how vitamin deficiencies can affect the skin and in some cases these translate also to the human being.

VITAMIN A

The skin does appear to be sensitive to vitamin A deficiency which can manifest itself as a hard, stippled skin known as toad skin. There may also be small, raised lesions that are hard and deeply pigmented in deficiency of this vitamin. There are many minor skin complaints like acne, eczema and psoriasis that respond in some cases to vitamin A treatment. This may be given orally or applied directly as an ointment to the afflicted area or both. The excellent response that has been obtained suggests that vitamin A deficiency, even a localised one, may be a factor in the development of these skin irritations.

VITAMIN C

Tiny haemorrhages beneath the skin, known as petechiae, that appear to be scattered over a wide area are characteristic of vitamin C deficiency. In addition, hardened pimples sometimes appear over the hair follicles of the calves and buttocks if body vitamin levels are low. The hairs too are affected, taking on a spiral shape or failing to appear.

VITAMIN E

The development of unsightly scars and striae (stretch marks) may be a feature of mild vitamin E deficiency since such skin problems have been overcome or prevented by taking vitamin E orally and by applying the vitamin in a cream or ointment base directly to the affected skin.

VITAMIN K

Purple patches under the skin, known as purpura, may reflect a blood-clotting problem. Vitamin K is necessary for the normal clotting of blood and a deficiency may present with purple patches. Self-treatment of this condition is usually dietary since the vitamin is not usually available on general sale.

VITAMIN B COMPLEX

Adequate intakes of all these vitamins are needed for a healthy skin, so not surprisingly, this tissue is amongst the first to be affected by even a mild deficiency. When pyridoxine (vitamin B6) is lacking the result is a dry, scaly skin with an excessive looseness resulting in a loss of body hair. The condition of seborrhoea, induced by an excessive secretion of the sebaceous glands of the skin, is seen about the eyes, nose, lips and mouth, sometimes extending to the eyebrows and ears, when pyridoxine intakes are low. Other obvious signs are redness of the moist surfaces of the body; a scaly and pigmented dermatitis is often seen around the neck, forearms, elbows and thighs.

Deficiency of riboflavin (vitamin B2) produces typical skin lesions manifested, in the main, by cracking of the lips and cracks in the corners of the mouth, the condition known as Cheilosis. Dermatitis, characterised by a red, itchy skin with the development of small blisters, is often a feature of riboflavin deficiency particularly in the areas of the nose, lips and genitals. Ulcers may appear on the lips and wet surfaces of the body.

Gross deficiency of nicotinic acid or nicotinamide (vitamin B3) leads to the serious disease pellagra, one of the characteristics of which is a rough, horny skin. This starts with a temporary redness, rather like sunburn, which clears to produce a more severe coloration in the form of deep red spots. These coalesce to form a dark, red or purple eruption followed by scaling and loss of skin, the areas most affected are the face, neck, hands and feet – on the hands the condition is called 'pellagrous glove'. Milder deficiency of the vitamin can also produce similar skin problems, not perhaps to the same extent, but characteristic nevertheless.

Pantothenic acid (vitamin B5) deficiency can produce 'burning feet' sensations on the soles where the skin feels to be hot and sore and it is difficult to put the foot down. Some of the skin symptoms associated with riboflavin deficiency may also clear up with pantothenic acid therapy, suggesting that they are a result of a lack of both vitamins. When pantothenic acid is lacking in some animals, skin ulceration and greying of hair result. Human beings do not usually show such signs but occasionally both have responded to supplementary pantothenic acid.

In infants, deficiency of the B vitamin biotin produces a localised, scaly, shedding dermatitis that responds only to this vitamin. Adults are less likely to suffer a similar skin condition due to biotin deficiency because the bacteria that inhabit the lower end of the intestine produce ample quantities of the vitamin. Infants may have a population of intestinal bacteria which has not developed enough to avail themselves of this facility.

The Mouth

Although we shall deal with how lack of individual vitamins affects the mouth, the symptoms may be more indicative of a generalised deficiency and treatment of oral lesion is usually best dealt with by the whole of the vitamin B complex and vitamin C. When riboflavin is lacking the first signs are a sore tongue with cracking of the lips and of the angles of the mouth, usually accompanied by intractable mouth ulcers. The tongue takes on a characteristic magenta colour with deep fissures and raised areas known as papillae.

In nicotinic acid deficiency the tongue will be swollen and the colour of raw beef. Other parts of the mouth affected include the gums, the mouth and the tongue, all of which become inflamed. An inflamed tongue may also be indicative of pyridoxine deficiency but in other respects, lack of the vitamin causes cracking of the lips and of the corners of the mouth – conditions also associated with low intakes of riboflavin.

The smooth, sore tongue associated with vitamin B12 deficiency is almost diagnostic of the condition. An inability to absorb the vitamin may give rise to pernicious anaemia. This serious complaint will only respond to vitamin B12 and treatment is only by intramuscular injection of the vitamin. A generalised low dietary intake of vitamin B12 now common in vegetarians and particularly vegans, will usually affect the tongue early on in the deficiency and healing is rapid once the vitamin is supplied in the diet.

Although we tend to associate disorders of the mouth and tongue with a possible vitamin B complex deficiency, lack of vitamin C is also a likely cause of such lesions. In low vitamin C intakes there are bleeding gums, which can become inflamed, leading to a loosening of the teeth. Small localised haemorrhages may also appear in the mouth. As we saw above, biotin deficiency is more likely in the infant because of its immature intestinal bacterial population. When the specific skin dermatitis appears, this may continue into the mouth, causing rawness on its surface. The condition will respond only to biotin.

The Gastro-Intestinal Tract

The digestive system can be affected by vitamin B complex deficiency at any level. Diarrhoea can be due to many causes but it is also a feature of thiamine or nicotinic acid deficiency. If thiamine is lacking, the diarrhoea is usually accompanied by abdominal distension and stomach pains. In the absence of any other obvious cause of persistent diarrhoea, the possibility of a vitamin B complex deficiency should always be considered and the appropriate therapy started.

Pantothenic acid deficiency has been shown to cause temporary paralysis of the intestinal tract, particularly when this occurs in the post-operative state. The condition is known as paralytic ileus and it is characterised by abdominal distress and distension, sometimes with the inability to pass motions. It is, therefore, a sensible precaution to ensure the body levels of pantothenic acid are adequate in the period before undergoing an abdominal operation, to reduce the chances of developing paralytic ileus.

The Eyes

When certain vitamins are lacking, both the process of sight and the health of the eye tissues can be adversely affected. Night blindness is a specific symptom of vitamin A deficiency that is characterised by poor adaptation of the eyes to low-intensity light conditions. Vision is normal under bright daylight or artificial light conditions but is lost in the dark. In the absence of the vitamin eye tissues also become abnormal – they are dry and thickened, particularly in the cornea or white of the eye and in the conjunctiva or wet membrane of the eye.

The white of the eye is also affected by riboflavin deficiency – it becomes bloodshot due to minute haemorrhages of the blood vessels. Other features are conjunctivitis or inflammation of the wet membranes particularly in the lower eyelid; a feeling of grittiness in the eye; a constant watering of the eye. Failing vision may occur if the deficiency worsens.

Thiamine (vitamin B1) deficiency is most likely to give rise to a dimness of vision that cannot be associated with a specific condition of the eye.

The eye muscles too are affected by low levels of the vitamin. There are often involuntary rhythmic movements of the eyeballs, known as nystagmus, fatigue of the eye muscles and paralysis of the eye resulting in reduced clearness of vision. Similar lesions are seen in nicotinic acid deficiency; which suggests that they may be associated more with a generalised vitamin B complex lack rather than a specific one.

Haemorrhages inside the eye often appear in vitamin C deficiency before they are obvious on the skin. Similarly when vitamin K levels are low, as in new-born babies, the first signs are haemorrhages in the retina of the eye. Similar lesions are observed in adults also, but deficiency of the vitamin is more likely in the new-born. This is because vitamin K does not readily pass across the placenta from mother to child and the intestinal bacteria of the new-born are not developed sufficiently to supply the vitamin from that source. Hence, as in the case of the B vitamin biotin, the new-born baby is also at risk of vitamin K deficiency.

The Central Nervous System

The normal metabolism of the nerves and brain depends upon adequate intakes of all the members of the vitamin B complex. Hence, deficiency of one or more of these vitamins will give rise to symptoms affecting the nervous system. When thiamine levels are low, mental confusion results leading eventually to coma. Milder deficiency causes involuntary rhythmic movement of the eyeballs (nystagmus) and this is one of the first signs. Other obvious mental symptoms include confabulation (narration of exaggerated fictitional experiences) and a generalised nerve inflammation that results in foot and wrist drop, due to lack of nervous control of the appropriate muscles.

When pyridoxine is low in infants the consequence is often the appearance of convulsions. This is because the vitamin is essential in the production of the brain substance GABA (gamma aminobutyric acid), which normally has a calming effect upon brain function. When it is lacking, control is lost and convulsions result. In adults, lack of pyridoxine more often manifests itself in mild depression and in generalised inflammation of the nerves, leading to tingling, numbness, burning pain and loss of vibratory sensation.

A similar generalised inflammation of the nerves is an early feature of nicotinic acid deficiency, but, in addition, an inflammatory condition of brain, known as encephalopathy, also appears. This becomes worse as the deficiency develops further, leading to a progressive dementia characterised by apprehension, confusion, derangement and maniacal outbursts.

Although the first detectable sign of vitamin B12 deficiency is often anaemia, a progressive nervous degeneration eventually manifests itself. The symptoms are pins and needles in the feet and hands, weakness in the limbs, stiffness in the legs leading to unsteadiness, lethargy and easy fatigue. In advanced deficiency, mental confusion and delirium are often seen, particularly in the aged. Reflexes are depressed leading to slow reactions and there is often an impairment of the sensation of touch. The tragedy is that although the anaemia associated with vitamin B12 deficiency is readily reversed by injection of the vitamin, a stage in nervous degeneration can be reached which is irreversible. Because of this, if any of the symptoms mentioned above appear, it is absolutely essential that professional diagnosis and treatment of the condition of vitamin B12 deficiency is undertaken at the earliest opportunity.

When folic acid is deficient in the body, the only mental symptom likely to be encountered is mental derangement whereby the individual is confused and lacks the ability to describe events, and is unaware of any abnormality. Professional guidance is essential to distinguish between folic acid and vitamin B12 deficiencies since correct diagnosis is essential before the appropriate therapy can be undertaken.

The Blood

Deficiencies of vitamins can also induce changes in other parts of the body. Unlike those discussed above, which may be obvious to the individual, these other changes are usually detected only in clinical examinations. The blood is amongst those tissues affected by the lack of specific vitamins which can result in anaemia of various types. Symptoms of anaemia, of whatever type, are similar and include paleness, tiredness, lethargy, breathlessness, weakness, vertigo, headache, constant noises in the head (tinnitus), spots before the eyes, drowsiness, irritability, cessation of periods, loss of libido and sometimes low-grade fever. Occasionally, there are gastro-intestinal complaints, and even heart failure can develop.

Correct treatment of the particular type of anaemia requires correct diagnosis which must be left to the medical practitioner. However, by looking to your intake of the vitamins required to prevent anaemia, you can at least ensure against developing the condition which is induced by their deficiency.

When the red blood cells are depleted of the oxygen-carrying substance known as haemoglobin the resulting condition is called hypochromic anaemia. Sometimes the red blood cells are also smaller than usual, when the condition is known as microcytic hypochromic anaemia. This type of anaemia may be caused by a deficiency of either pyridoxine or riboflavin or even both. Megaloblastic anaemia is of a completely different type where the red blood cells are deprived of haemoglobin and are irregular in size. Lots of immature red blood cells, which are not capable of carrying oxygen, also appear in the blood. The most likely cause of megaloblastic anaemia is a lack of vitamin B12 or folic acid, or of both vitamins.

The most common type of anaemia is that due to iron deficiency. Iron occupies an essential, central role in haemoglobin – in fact oxygen is carried on the back of the iron in haemoglobin. Iron cannot be absorbed from the food or from supplements without vitamin C, so deficiency of this vitamin may also give rise to iron-deficient anaemia. At the same time in the absence of vitamin C, iron cannot be incorporated into the haemoglobin protein. Lack of vitamin C, as we have seen, can also cause loss of blood through haemorrhage so this too can contribute to the development of anaemia. Even when iron is adequate in the diet, unless it is accompanied by sufficient vitamin C, it cannot be efficiently absorbed and utilised. In fact, many researchers believe that if we all had adequate intakes of vitamin C, we would all make better use of the iron in our diets even when intake of the mineral was low.

Lack of vitamin E in the blood can give rise to what is known as haemolytic anaemia. In this condition the red blood cells are weakened to such an extent that they burst easily, spilling their content of haemoglobin into the blood. Once haemoglobin has left the red blood cell it no longer has the capacity to carry oxygen. Hence, if too many red blood cells burst, the oxygen-carrying function of the blood is severely reduced and symptoms of anaemia result. Adequate vitamin E intakes will prevent haemolytic anaemia by toughening up the membranes of the red blood cells which hold them together.

The Heart and Blood Vessels

Thiamine deficiency in the later stages causes severely weakened heart muscle which can lead to heart failure. Gross enlargement of the heart is also a feature of thiamine deficiency. A different effect upon the heart and blood vessels is manifested by pyridoxine deficiency. Massive fat deposits are laid down in the walls of these organs, leading to the condition, known as atherosclerosis, which severely restricts the flow of blood. As the insidious process continues, the ultimate result is complete deprivation of blood, and hence oxygen, to the heart muscle itself when heart failure is inevitable.

The Bones

Pain in the bones can be related to some vitamin deficiencies but as the condition can also be due to other factors, diagnosis of the cause of bone pain is best left to the medical practitioner who can enlist the aid of X-rays and other techniques. Nevertheless, vitamin C in high doses has been used to reduce bone pain. Lack of vitamin D, in both adults and children, can cause bone problems which will respond only to treatment with the vitamin. As the deficiency in most of these cases is simply lack of dietary vitamin D, sometimes combined with deprivation of sunlight on the body, the remedy is obvious – ensure the diet contains vitamin D-rich foods and try to spend some time out in the fresh air. The conditions induced by low vitamin D intakes are rickets in children and osteomalacia in adults.

The Reproductive System

Most of our knowledge on the effect of vitamin deficiencies on the reproductive system of both males and females has come from animal studies. The two most important vitamins in this respect are B12 and E although recent reports suggest that lack of vitamin C can cause less fertile male spermatozoa. In the male of the species, lack of these vitamins causes decreased production and mobility of the sperm leading, in extreme deficiency, to sterility. In the female, conception is still possible when intakes of these vitamins are low, but the offspring rarely reach full term. There are scattered reports that both vitamin E and B12 have helped some couples to conceive when their previous inability to do so was due to mild deficiency of the vitamins. However, there is a lack of hard evidence that vitamin deficiency plays a major role in causing sterility and infertility in people, despite some small success with vitamin therapy and the fact that animals have a need for adequate vitamin intake for full reproductive capacity.

We have seen in this chapter how self-examination or the observation of others can give a clue to possible deficiencies of specific vitamins in the body. The reasons why we may not be getting our full complement of these essential micro nutrients are many and varied. The choice of food; the way it is cooked, processed and stored; the amount eaten are all contributory factors in determining vitamin intake. In addition, lifestyles, social habits, diseases, pregnancy, medicinal drugs and other stresses may increase daily requirements of vitamins, often to levels above those that can be obtained even in an excellent diet. Little wonder then that many individuals existing on barely adequate intakes of vitamins will develop deficiency symptoms when their circumstances change under the influence of the factors mentioned above.

SUMMARY TABLE
Signs and Symptoms of Vitamin Deficiency

Affected Area	Signs/Symptoms	Possible Vitamin Deficiency
General	Fatigue, malaise, apathy, depression	Usually B complex
	Loss of appetite	Vitamin B1, vitamin B12
Nervous System	Headache	Vitamin B6, niacinamide
	Tingling, numbness, burning skin	Vitamin B1, vitamin B2
	Low back pain	Folic acid, vitamin B12
	Lack of muscular co-ordination	Vitamin B1, vitamin B12
	Personality changes	Niacinamide
	Loss of memory	Vitamin B1, vitamin B12 niacinamide, folic acid
	Muscle wasting and weakness	Vitamin B1, vitamin B6
	Loss of senses	Vitamin B1, vitamin B6
	Dragging of the feet (footdrop)	Vitamin B1
	Reduced tendon jerks	Vitamin B1
	Sub acute combined degeneration of the spinal cord	Vitamin B12
	Stress	Vitamin B Complex, vitamin C, vitamin E
Skin	Haemorrhaging	Vitamin C, vitamin K
	Dry skin	Vitamin A
	Yellow colouration	Vitamin B12
	Hardening of the skin	Vitamin A
	Spiral and unerupted hairs	Vitamin C
	Genitalia dermatitis	Vitamin B2, niacinamide
	Burning feet	Pantothenic acid
	Pallor	Folic acid, vitamin B12
	Scar tissue	Vitamin E
	Pregnancy striae	Vitamin E
Eyes	Poor night vision	Vitamin A
	Dry eyes	Vitamin A, vitamin B2
	Blurred vision	Vitamin B1
	Bloodshot eyes	Vitamin B2
	Dim vision	Vitamin B1, niacinamide
	Intraocular haemorrhage	Vitamin C, vitamin K
	Optic neuritis	Vitamin B1, vitamin B12

SUMMARY TABLE *continued*
Signs and Symptoms of Vitamin Deficiency

Affected Area	*Signs/Symptoms*	*Possible Vitamin Deficiency*
Lips, tongue and mouth	Inflammation	Vitamin B2
	Ulceration	Vitamin B2
	Fissures at corners of lips	Vitamin B2, vitamin B6
	Lips that hurt	Vitamin B1
	Sore tongue, inflamed tongue	Vitamin B12, vitamin B2, Niacinamide, folic acid, vitamin B6
	Beefy red swollen tongue	Niacinamide
	Fissured tongue	Vitamin B2
	Magenta-coloured	Vitamin B2
Gums	Bleeding and spongy	Vitamin C
	Gingivitis (inflamed)	Niacinamide
Face	Seborrhoea of nose and lips	Vitamin B2, vitamin B6
	Cheek pigmentation	Niacinamide
Skeletal system	Softening of the skull (babies)	Vitamin D
	Swelling of the skull (babies)	Vitamin D .
	Swelling of the joints (babies)	Vitamin D
	Painful bleeding of joints	Vitamin C
Gastrointestinal	Diarrhoea	Niacinamide
	Digestive disorders	Vitamin B1
	Paralytic ileus	Pantothenic acid
Blood	Anaemia	Folic acid, vitamin B12 vitamin C, vitamin B6
	Haemolytic anaemia	Vitamin E

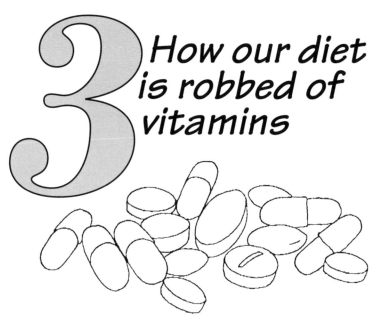

3 How our diet is robbed of vitamins

Having established that our food as provided by nature contains all the vitamins we need for health, let us look now how those vitamins can be depleted by the way we treat our food from the time it is picked or butchered, to when it is eaten.

Storage and processing

Simply storing vegetables can give rise to serious losses of vitamin C. Potatoes, for example, when freshly dug from the ground will contain about 30mg of vitamin C per 100g (3.5oz). After three months storage, in the dark and at ordinary temperatures, this level has dropped to 20mg per 100g; after five months it is only 15mg per 100g; after seven months it is reduced to 10mg per 100g; after nine months only 8mg vitamin C is left in 100g potatoes. To many people potatoes represent the main source of their daily vitamin C intake and when these are old, as in the spring months before the new crops appear their contribution of vitamin C is minimal. This is the reason why some old people, particularly in low income groups and where fruit is perceived as expensive, develop symptoms of abject scurvy during the month of

April. Once the new potatoes appear and are eaten they contain enough vitamin C to cure the condition until months later when, after the vitamin has been depleted in the stored vegetables, the deficiency cycle starts again.

Even storage of foods at refrigeration, or freezer temperatures, can lead to substantial losses. Vitamin E is lost readily at deep freeze temperatures of −12°C. Potato crisps, for example, which can supply useful amounts of the vitamin from the vegetable oil in which they are cooked (although they are generally thought to be of low nutritional value and are usually termed junk food), will lose 68 percent and 74 percent of their vitamin E after storage at −12°C for periods of one month and two months respectively. The B vitamin pantothenic acid disappears slowly from all types of food that are kept frozen.

Air and light are the greatest natural destroyers of vitamins. Riboflavin is readily converted into a compound called lumiflavin by the action of light. Unfortunately, lumiflavin in turn destroys vitamin C. Hence, if milk is left for long periods in sunlight or even under shop lights not only does the riboflavin disappear but vitamin C losses are also substantial.

Milk remains one of our more important sources of riboflavin so such losses can be serious. Milk should, therefore, be transferred to a refrigerator as soon as possible after delivery or collection to preserve its vitamin content. Other vitamins that are readily broken down by light include A, carotene and B12.

Some vitamins are readily oxidised and hence destroyed by the action of the oxygen in the air. Whilst many storage conditions exclude air, it is easy to inadvertently destroy vitamin C, for example, by commonplace practices. Fruit juices and drinks are often taken for their vitamin C content but this can be reduced rapidly once the container has been opened. Studies have indicated that orange drink preparations lost between 30 and 50 percent of their vitamin content within eight days of opening a sealed bottle; after three to four weeks 90 percent had been lost. Losses were accelerated by shaking the bottles vigorously – a practice that is common amongst consumers. The vitamin C in apple juice is lost even more rapidly. 50 percent was lost after four days; 95 percent was destroyed after only 16 days storage at the relatively low temperature of 5°C, which is lower than the average domestic refrigerator. Fruit and vegetable juices are a pleasant and convenient way of taking vitamin C, but there is little to be gained by storing them for long periods once the container is opened. Careful decanting from the container will also help to preserve the vitamin from the destructive action of air.

All fruit and vegetables lose vitamins when stored at ambient temperatures. Some are preserved to a large extent by storing at deep freeze temperatures and this must be regarded as the best way to retain food for long periods. Do not forget however that before freezing, vegetables are blanched and this process can contribute to losses of vitamins even before the food is frozen. The best way to maintain the vitamin potency of food is to eat it as fresh as possible and avoid long periods of storage. If it must be stored, keep it at deep freeze temperatures.

The drying of some foods can also adversely affect certain vitamins. Dried vegetables and fruits lose virtually all of their vitamin C during the drying process but the B vitamins at least survive in the main. Freeze-drying represents the least destructive method of removing water but for most foods this process has not yet reached commercial levels.

Carotene losses in vegetables and fruits range from 10-20 percent under controlled, mild conditions of drying to virtually complete destruction in traditional open-air drying. Storage losses of both vitamin A and carotene can be substantial in certain foods even at refrigerator temperatures. Butter loses up to 30 percent of its vitamin A content after twelve months at 5°C; at higher room temperatures (as in the tropics) losses are 35 percent after only five months. For some reason, vitamin A and carotene are far more stable in margarines – possibly because of the differing fatty acid contents. Similarly, destruction of vitamin A is minimal in skimmed milk powder after three months even at blood temperatures but serious losses occur after twelve months.

The critical time for both vegetable foods and those of animal origin appears to be about three months. It is only after this time that losses start to become significant. Hence any storage beyond this time can seriously affect the vitamin A and carotene contents of all foods. Remember that these periods are measured from the time of manufacture so that when the foods reach your refrigerator their shelf life could already have been some weeks. The existence of 'butter mountains' in the EEC community and the relatively slow turnover of this foodstuff is likely to render the product virtually devoid of these vitamins once it reaches the consumer.

Don't imagine that all the vitamins in raw foodstuffs start disappearing once the food has left the ground or the tree because vitamins vary widely in their stability. Vitamins B2, C and E are particularly susceptible in this respect but the remainder of the vitamin B complex will still be there when the food is eaten or cooked. Bruising of vegetables and fruits is particularly harmful to these unstable vitamins because it breaks down cells within the structure of the fruit and vegetable. Enzymes are released and these can have a destructive effect upon the micronutrients. Within the intact cell everything is kept in order and separated by intercell partitioning so there is no chance of interaction. Once cell walls are broken the contents mix and the introduction of air accelerates destruction of the vitamins. Intact food substances have a stabilising effect upon vitamins as they protect them from light and air. It is only bad handling and storage, combined with destructive cooking methods, which bring about a decline in the level of vitamins present in food.

The refining and processing of basic foodstuffs can also contribute to loss and destruction of some vitamins. For an example we need look no further than the refining of wholemeal flour to the popular white variety. All the vitamins present in wholemeal or wholewheat flour are reduced drastically when refined into white flour. These losses are so serious that government legislation forces millers to put back thiamine and nicotinic acid into white flour. Even with this fortification, however, the levels of thiamine and nicotinic acid in white flour are 32.6 percent and 64.3 percent lower respectively than in the wholemeal type. Unfortunately, the drastic reductions in other vitamins content that result from the refining of flour are not redressed so white flour and the products made from it are grossly depleted of vitamins.

Similar losses of vitamins are encountered when raw cane sugar is converted into the pure white variety. Hence what is a useful food with its full complement of vitamins and minerals as supplied by nature becomes simply a source of calories only – an 'empty calorie' food. Rice too is virtually depleted of its vitamins when it is refined from the raw, unpolished natural variety into the more popular but less nutritious white rice. Dried potato products often have added vitamin C but this is only a replacement for the natural material destroyed during the drying process.

Fat soluble vitamins too are lost by food refining – the vitamin E in wholegrain wheat is neatly disposed of during the production of white flour. Serious losses also occur when cooking oils are extracted from grains, seeds and beans since vitamin E does not stand up to the solvents and heating applied during their extraction. Vitamin A, and Carotene particularly, do survive most refining processes as long as light is excluded.

The reasons why refining certain wholefoods causes wholesale loss of vitamins are twofold. First, as in the case of grains and rice, the portion disposed of, like the bran, is the main source of vitamins and of minerals. Second, the methods used in refining are often destructive because of the applications of heat and solvents, etc. At least in the first case the vitamins can be reclaimed by utilizing the part removed, like the bran or wheatgerm. In the second case they are lost forever.

The losses we have discussed above have usually occurred before the food has reached our kitchens. Let us now look at how cooking processes can also contribute to a depletion of vitamins. In addition, we shall see how a little thought and trouble can retain these essential micronutrients during the cooking of food, at least when under our control in the kitchen.

How vitamins are lost in cooking

Most of the food we eat is cooked, either by ourselves in the kitchen, or in a factory by a food manufacturer, or in a take-away fast food supplier. The act of cooking itself can cause losses of vitamins from that food but there are distinct differences in how we can control those losses. In the kitchen, cooking losses can be regained to a large extent; when the food is prepared elsewhere the lost vitamins are gone forever. Food losses of vitamins during cooking processes are a combination of partial destruction of these sensitive micronutrients and those amounts that are leached out into the cooking fluids. We can limit the actual destruction of vitamins but can't do much about them once they are gone. Leached vitamins can be recovered. Fortunately, in most domestic cooking processes, the losses due to leaching far outweigh the quantities irreversibly destroyed. The factors that determine the extent of cooking losses of vitamins during cooking are:

1. The method of cooking.

2. The time of cooking.

3. The temperature of cooking.

4. The volume of water or of cooking fat in which the food is cooked.

5. The physical state of the food being cooked.

In boiling vegetables, for example, the highest losses are associated with a large volume of boiling water, a prolonged boiling time, and finely divided vegetables. Both carotene and vitamin E, because they are fat-soluble, are not affected by the boiling process, irrespective of whether the vegetable is the root kind, the leafy type or is a seed, e.g. peas, beans. All the watersoluble vitamins, i.e. the vitamin B complex and C, are lost to a certain extent when these types of vegetables are boiled, usually between 30 and 50 percent of the original content. Fortunately, most of these losses are simply leaching into the boiling water so they can be recovered by utilizing that water.

VITAMIN C

This is the most unstable of the vitamins and its losses during cooking processes can be quite substantial.

The proportion of losses due to destruction and those due to leaching is from 10 percent to 55 percent and from less than 10 percent to 60 percent respectively. Steaming and pressure cooking of green vegetables and of root vegetables destroy from 20 to 40 percent of the vitamin C present but the percentage lost by leaching is less than 10 percent. The reverse occurs in simple boiling of these vegetables.

The other water-soluble vitamins behave in a similar fashion. If the cooking water is utilized in some way, the percentage of vitamin C available to the body increases to 60-90 in all cases.

These figures apply only to a once-cooked vegetable. If this is stored then re-heated at a later date, losses are much more substantial and in some cases virtually all the vitamin is destroyed. There is a classic case on record of a children's hospital in Vienna where 40 out of 64 children who were long-stay patients, developed scurvy because of the practice of feeding them re-heated vegetables. These vegetables were boiled in bulk for long periods; the water was discarded; the boiled vegetables were set aside and re-heated at daily intervals. Little wonder that their vitamin C content turned out to be virtually zero!

Beware, too, of another common practice, especially where large quantities of foods are prepared in advance. Potatoes and other root vegetables when soaked overnight in cold water will lose up to 60 percent of their vitamin C content by leaching into the water. If the water is discarded most of the original vitamin C will accompany it down the drain. Similarly, machine peeling of vegetables is more destructive to the vitamin C than the hand process. This then is another practice associated with large scale, institutional preparation of foods that leads to wholesale losses of vitamin C and the other water-soluble vitamins.

Not surprisingly, the large-leafed vegetables, like cabbage, which present a high surface area to the boiling water are the more likely to lose their vitamin C by leaching. Boiling cabbage for 20 minutes reduced its vitamin C content by 70 percent; simmering it at 70 to 80°C for 60 minutes reduced it by 90 percent. Fortunately, the vitamin can be recovered in the main by using the water to make a sauce, or gravy, or in some other way.

Root vegetables, like potatoes, will lose more vitamin C if they are diced than if they are cooked whole. The following losses in potatoes are those expected with the appropriate cooking technique mentioned; peeled, boiled then mashed 30 to 50 percent; unpeeled boiled 20 to 40 percent; baked 20 to 40 percent; roast 20 to 40 percent; steamed 20 to 40 percent; chipped 25 to 35 percent lost. This means that new potatoes subjected to these methods will supply between 18 and 24mg vitamin C per 100g (3.5 oz.) as eaten. When the potatoes are old, they will provide only between 4.8 and 6.4mg vitamin C per 100g. This is not sufficient to supply even the minimum daily quantity needed to prevent the deficiency disease scurvy.

The B Vitamins

THIAMINE

Amongst the B vitamins, thiamine (vitamin B1) is the least stable which may explain why, according to the World Health Organisation, this vitamin is the one most likely to be deficient in diets worldwide. It is stable only under acid conditions, which means that any alkaline treatment of foods containing the vitamin will destroy most of it. Trace minerals, like copper, present in some cooking utensils, will accelerate the destruction of thiamine. Sulphur dioxide, widely used to preserve foodstuffs, completely inactivates the vitamin.

This preservative is often added to mince both to prolong the shelf-life of the meat and to maintain its attractive red colour. Forty-eight hours after treating mince with sulphur dioxide, the thiamine content is reduced by 90 percent. You should therefore avoid sulphur dioxide treated meats if you wish to preserve your intake of thiamine. Similarly, beware of ready-peeled potatoes which are kept white by adding sulphite solution (i.e. sulphur dioxide in water). This treatment will dispose of about 55 percent of the thiamine originally present in the potatoes. As these vegetables are the only ones that contribute significant quantities of thiamine to the diet, using preserved or commercially processed potatoes as the main source of the vegetable, will add insignificant amounts of the vitamin and lead to the development of deficiency.

Although you must be aware of losses of thiamine in cooking processes, in good quality foods the protein and amino acids present will help protect the vitamin. Starches also assist in the absorption of thiamine. This is why cereals, which contain both protein and starch, are added to tinned meats, particularly those containing pork which represents a very rich source of thiamine. Cereals are thus excellent natural preservatives of the thiamine in cooked meats.

Apart from destruction of the vitamin by processing methods often carried out before you buy the food, the principal losses of thiamine are due to its water solubility. The more finely divided or ground the food is, the greater the loss. Chopped and minced foods can lose from 20 to 70 percent of their thiamine but it can be recovered by eating the extracted liquors. When meat is cooked at 150°C there is virtually no destruction of the vitamin but there are considerable losses into the exuded juices, although these can be recovered of course. At temperatures of 200°C however, at least 20 percent of the thiamine is destroyed. Over-cooking of meat should therefore be avoided if you wish to preserve its thiamine content.

The instability of thiamine in alkaline substances is illustrated nicely by observing its losses from boiled rice. When pure, distilled water is used, losses are nil. Tap water which is slightly alkaline causes 8 to 10 percent loss; the more alkaline well water gives rise to 36 percent loss.

Simple baking processes cause 15 to 25 percent destruction of thiamine, but when baking powder is added (this is highly alkaline) at least half the vitamin is destroyed.

When bread is baked, between 15 and 30 percent of the thiamine content of the flour is destroyed. Most of the destruction takes place in the crust so the popular practice of removing this part of the bread before eating it is not laying one open to B1 deficiency. Remember, that further losses of thiamine will result when the bread is toasted. Light toast is to be preferred to the darker variety if you wish to minimise thiamine losses.

Meats represent a very important source of thiamine in the diet so losses encountered in the various ways of cooking it can vary from 30 to 80 percent with roasting and braising being the least destructive processes. Remember, however, to utilize the various juices that are produced during these cooking methods if you want to ensure the maximum intake of thiamine. If the meat you cook has been frozen, be sure to utilize the liquids dripped during the thawing – these are rich sources of leached vitamin B 1. In the canned variety, use of the juices recovers lost vitamins.

Thiamine losses from fish also depend upon the cooking method used, e.g. percentage losses are poaching, 10; baking, 30; frying, 40; grilling, 20. In some countries, notably Japan, raw fish represents an important item of food but when eaten uncooked, thiamine can be lost. The reason is that raw fish contains an enzyme called thiaminase which destroys thiamine whilst the food is in the gastro-intestinal system. Normal cooking methods will destroy thiaminase but this of course survives if the fish is eaten raw. There are many cases on record of thiamine deficiency, sometimes leading to beriberi, in Japanese who eat large amounts of raw fish.

Losses of thiamine during the cooking of vegetables depends largely on the type of vegetable. Root vegetables will lose 25 percent; leafy vegetables will lose 40 percent; seeds lose 30 percent. Milk is a useful source of thiamine but losses can occur during the various processing methods as the following percentage losses show: pasteurization 10; sterilisation 20; UHT 10; boiling 0.

RIBOFLAVIN

The vitamin (also known as B2) is stable to air, acid and heat up to 130°C. The most destructive elements are alkalis and light. Because of its water solubility, riboflavin is readily lost by leaching from chopped foods in wet processing and cooking methods.

Light must be excluded if the riboflavin in foodstuffs is to be preserved, particularly in liquid foods like milk. Even a relatively low level of destruction of riboflavin to the product lumiflavin (5 percent) can cause 50 percent of the vitamin C content to be destroyed by the action of the lumiflavin. Studies indicate that milk exposed to light in summer loses 90 percent of its riboflavin content in full sunshine in 2 hours; 45 percent in cloudy weather; 30 percent when the sky is completely clouded over. Room lighting causes 30 percent loss within 24 hours. Bread, too, is affected by light. Supermarket lighting destroyed 17 percent of the riboflavin content of bread rolls in 24 hours; 13 percent when the rolls were wrapped in amber plastic film; 2 percent when wrapped in orange plastic.

Although riboflavin is perfectly stable in cold storage beef when light is excluded, losses can occur once it is cooked. 20 percent is lost during the roasting, frying and grilling of meats and poultry; 30 percent is lost when meat and poultry is stewed or boiled. Similarly, whilst the vitamin is stable in raw, fresh fish, percentage losses during the following cooking processes are: poaching 0; baking 20; frying or grilling 20. When vegetables are cooked percentage losses of riboflavin are 30 (root-type); 40 (leafy-type); 30 (seed-type). When possible, therefore, it is wise to eat vegetables raw to ensure the maximum intake of riboflavin. When this is not possible, as for example in certain seeds and pulses, the losses induced by cooking can be counteracted by eating the cooking fluids.

Milk and meats represent our most important sources of dietary riboflavin. Cold milk that has had the minimum exposure to light is an excellent food in this respect but boiling it will reduce the riboflavin content by between 12 and 25 percent. Pasteurized milk will have lost about 14 percent of its riboflavin content when it reaches you but the rest of the vitamin can be preserved by taking the precautions in storing mentioned above. Dry or wet curing of meats will cause 40 percent loss in riboflavin level so this should be taken into account and regarded as additional to further losses induced by various cooking methods.

NICOTINIC ACID

This is the most stable of the B complex of vitamins so losses in cooking are mainly a result of leaching. The vitamin is unaffected by heat, air, light, acidity, alkalinity and by sulphite or sulphur dioxide. There are losses of 20 percent of the nicotinic acid content of meats and poultry when they are roasted, fried or grilled; and of 50 percent when these foodstuffs are stewed or boiled. Fish will lose 10 percent when poached and 20 percent when baked, fried or grilled. Root vegetables and seeds will lose 30 percent of their nicotinic acid content when boiled; leafy vegetables will lose 40 percent. All of these losses can be recovered and made available to the diet simply by utilizing the cooking water of juices. Remember too, that some will be lost into the thawed drippings, from frozen foods but these also are recoverable.

Nicotinic acid is unique amongst the vitamins in that it can be liberated from certain foods by the cooking process. This is because in cereals the vitamin is bound to starches and proteins in a complex called niacytin. This complex is resistant to digestion by the normal digestive processes of the body. In wheat flour, a significant 77 percent of its nicotinic acid content is present in this bound form. The best way to liberate the free nicotinic acid is to bake the flour with alkaline baking powder. In Mexico, maize (corn) is soaked overnight in lime water before using it to make the staple food tortillas. This practice makes the nicotinic acid content of maize available in the diet. It was a prime factor in ensuring that Mexican peasants did not suffer from nicotinic acid deficiency (a disease called "Pellagra") in the 1920's, when their USA counterparts over the border were dying from pellagra because their cooking techniques with the same raw food ingredients did not liberate the vitamin.

All the processing techniques used in milk and milk products and those utilizing eggs do not affect the nicotinic acid contents of these foods. Nor does the wet and dry curing of meats, apart from some leaching of the vitamin which is recoverable.

PYRIDOXINE

This B vitamin (B6) is stable in the presence of heat and indeed in most cooking methods. Acids and alkalis do not affect the vitamin but significant losses can occur in all cooking methods by leaching into cooking fluids, hence these can be recovered. The losses by leaching can be 20 percent during roasting, frying and grilling; 50 percent during stewing and boiling. Fish will lose no pyridoxine during poaching; but 10 percent is leached during baking and 20 percent during frying or grilling. When vegetables are boiled, losses in all types account for 40 percent of the original content of pyridoxine but the whole of the loss can be recovered by utilizing the boiling water because all losses are due to leaching. Canned foods also will contain much of their pyridoxine in the liquid portion so this too should be used to ensure maximum intakes of the vitamin. When thawing frozen foods prior to cooking, ensure the drips are re-introduced into the diet since these too contain pyridoxine. This is relatively simple with vegetables which tend to be dropped into boiling water but may not be so obvious when meat, poultry and fish are allowed to thaw for some hours.

The only food where significant destruction of pyridoxine can occur during processing is milk. This is because at high temperatures other components of milk will react with the vitamin causing its destruction. At one time, babies fed on milk treated by high temperature processing developed pyridoxine deficiency because of this loss. When modern methods of drying milk were developed the wholesale destruction of the vitamin ceased and the problem disappeared. However, it can still occur from time to time when over zealous parents process the milk for their offspring, using excessive temperatures.

FOLIC ACID

This B vitamin occurs in foods as the free vitamin and in various combination forms. Only the free form is unstable, mainly by oxidation. Sunlight, too, can be destructive and the action of light is accelerated by riboflavin. On the other hand, vitamin C exerts a protective effect. Despite this, 30 percent of the folic acid content of tomato juice is lost when this is stored in clear glass bottles; only 7 percent of the vitamin was lost from the juice stored in dark glass bottles.

Vegetables represent a very important source of folic acid in our diets and losses can be significant during cooking processes. For example, 10 percent is lost during steam blanching; 20 percent on pressure cooking; 25 to 50 percent on boiling. Again, some of these losses are due to leaching and so can be recovered. Sterilizing milk can give rise to losses varying from 20 to 100 percent, depending on the time of contact with the air.

There are cumulative losses of folic acid in food processing. Let us consider, for example, the canning of beans. Preliminary soaking for 12 hours will leach out 5 percent after 10 minutes and 45 percent after 20 minutes, only some of which is recoverable; final sterilization in the can will destroy 10 percent of that left. This means that very little folic acid will remain in the beans by the time they are eaten.

Losses from foods such as vegetables, fruits and dairy products average 70 percent of free folic acid and 45 percent of the total of free and conjugated varieties during the overall processes of cooking. The baking of bread will destroy some 30 percent of the folic acid present in the original flour, but the final content in wholemeal bread is higher than that in white bread.

These wholesale losses of folic acid during cooking processes make it imperative, therefore, that the diet where possible should contain fresh, raw vegetables, fruits and salads to provide the requirements of this vitamin. A complete reliance on cooked and processed foods will increase the chances of a mild deficiency, particularly during pregnancy where adequate intakes of folic acid are absolutely essential for the health of the growing, unborn child.

VITAMIN B12

This is stable under most conditions but it can be destroyed by alkalis. As the vitamin is protected by the proteins of the foodstuffs and as it is confined to foods of animal origins (which are high in protein) the chances of destruction during cooking are slight. Also, the daily requirements of vitamin B12 are so small it is highly unlikely that anyone eating meat and dairy products is going to develop deficiency because of losses during cooking procedures.

PANTOTHENIC ACID

A vitamin of the B group that is stable under most cooking methods that are carried out in neutral conditions, but some destruction can occur when acids and alkalis are present. Wheat, for example, can lose as much as 60 percent of its pantothenic acid content when baking powder is used during the manufacturing process of wheat products. Meats will lose 30 percent of their pantothenic acid content when cooked but most of this is leached out and so can be recovered. Losses during the storage of deep frozen meats can be as high as 8 percent, even at these low temperatures.

BIOTIN

This B vitamin has undergone very few studies on its stability during cooking processes. It is, however, produced in very significant quantities by the bacteria that inhabit the lower end of the intestine. In view of this source therefore the behaviour of biotin and its presence in foods during the various cooking procedures is probably of little significance. However 30 percent, most of which is recoverable, is lost during the boiling of vegetables; 10 percent lost during all methods of cooking fish; 10 percent is lost when meat and poultry are cooked by any method.

The Fat Soluble Vitamins

VITAMIN A

This vitamin and its precursor carotene are insoluble in water so they do not suffer losses through extraction into processing and cooking water. The main destructive agent is oxygen but in foods both vitamins A and carotene are protected by natural antioxidants like vitamin E.

Boiling water destroys 16 percent of the vitamin A content of margarine in 30 minutes; 40 percent in one hour and 70 percent in two hours. Frying is more destructive, with losses of 40 percent in 5 minutes; 60 percent in 10 minutes and 70 percent in 15 minutes. Braising liver causes up to 10 percent loss of its vitamin A content but the level is so high to start with that this loss is not significant.

Destruction of carotene occurs when green vegetables are cooked and they can lose between 15 and 20 percent of their vitamin A activity. (Carotene functions partly by being converted to vitamin A within the body so its activity is always expressed in terms of vitamin A). Yellow vegetables lose even more with losses of between 25 and 30 percent of their vitamin A activity after freezing or canning, followed by further cooking. This is significant because it was thought until recently that canned vegetables retained all their carotene content, even after many years. These losses therefore represent a conversion of the wholly active carotene in the original vegetable to a form that is less active.

The most significant losses, totalling between 10 and 20 percent, occur when fruits and vegetables are dried under mild conditions. Even these losses are greater when traditional open-air drying is carried out and virtually complete destruction can occur.

VITAMIN D

Vitamin D is regarded as being very stable but studies are few because of the difficulty of measuring the tiny amounts of the vitamin that occur in foods. Nevertheless, the vitamin has been found to withstand the smoking of fish, the pasteurization and sterilization of milk and the drying of eggs. There are probably losses of between 25 and 35 percent of vitamin D activity during the spray-drying of milk but this is allowed for in fortification of the food with the vitamin. The significance of food contents and losses during cooking processes of vitamin D is not clear because the vitamin is also produced by the action of sunlight on the skin. However, for those who are housebound or confined indoors for other reasons, the dietary intake of vitamin D is important to their daily requirements but it does look as though eating vitamin D-rich foods, cooked or otherwise, will supply their needs.

VITAMIN E

This is very sensitive to oxidation particularly in the presence of heat and alkalis. There are serious losses in frozen foods. The most significant losses, however, are the result of the processing and refining of cereals – a very important source. Cooking foods in fats destroys between 70 and 90 percent of the vitamin E content. Greatest losses occur in the presence of rancid fats and oils and, unfortunately, these cannot always be detected by taste. Continual use of the same cooking fats and oils (e.g. in the chip pan) progressively destroys the vitamins in the food being fried. It is a sensible idea to squirt the contents of a 1000mg capsule of vitamin E into the chip pan before using the oil for chip frying. This will at least ensure that the potatoes are protected against vitamin E loss while they are being fried. Don't put the whole capsule in as the gelatine coat will not dissolve in the oil. Make sure the vitamin E you add is natural d–alpha tocopherol since this is far more efficient than the synthetic dl–variety.

Boiling vegetables like sprouts, cabbage and carrots can destroy 30 percent of their vitamin E content. When vegetables are canned even greater losses of up to 80 percent can occur. Raw vegetables and nuts are exceptionally good sources of vitamin E, so make up for the cooking losses by ensuring that these feature in your diet.

Eggs are a rather special food since, unlike other foodstuffs mentioned above, eggs when cooked are unlikely to lose any vitamins by leaching. The rapid coagulation of the egg albumen protein during the cooking process tends to retain them all and, of course, when boiled the shell acts as a barrier. Losses are therefore all due to destruction of the vitamins and these can vary from 30 percent in fried eggs down to 10 percent in boiled of folic acid; 20 percent in fried down to 10 percent in boiled of thiamine; 20 percent in poached, scrambled or omelette down to 5 percent in boiled of riboflavine; 20 percent in fried down to 10% in boiled of pyridoxine and 20 percent in fried down to 10 percent in boiled of pantothenic acid. Amounts destroyed by poaching, scrambling or omelette are similar for all vitamins.

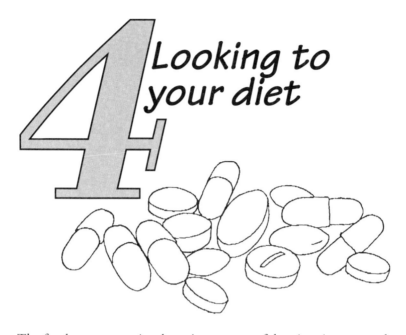

4 Looking to your diet

The food we eat remains the prime source of the vitamins we need and a careful selection of dietary items will ensure at least the minimum requirements of those essential micronutrients. This applies only under normal conditions of living however and as we shall see, lifestyles, habits, medicinal drugs, cooking methods, storage of food, digestive ability and many other factors can cause losses of vitamins or an increased body requirement. Self-help must therefore come first by considering the type of food we eat and the way we treat it before it is eaten. All natural food contains some vitamins and by eating a balanced mixture of food items a wide spectrum of vitamin intake will be obtained. Let us look, therefore, at the general principles of food levels of vitamins.

Dietary sources of vitamins

Cereals

These comprise an important part of the diet for their energy contribution to the body and for their dietary fibre content. They include grains, flours, starches, breakfast cereals, biscuits, cakes, buns, pastries and puddings. As cereal products tend to be eaten in large quantities their contribution of protein is also not insignificant. They supply excellent quantities of the vitamin B complex, apart from vitamin B12, but are completely devoid of vitamins A, D, C and the provitamin beta-carotene. Hence we must look to other food items to supply these missing vitamins

Despite the usefulness of cereals and cereal products as suppliers of the B vitamins (apart from B12) and indeed of vitamin E, the levels are reduced quite drastically by the refining and processing of the foods as provided by nature into the type that most of us eat. Whole grains and wholemeal flour represent the best unrefined cereals that we have in our diet, in the form of mueslis and wholemeal bread, which still retain their full complement of B vitamins (apart from vitamin B12) and vitamin E. Of course, when a wheatgrain is refined, the material removed such as the bran and wheatgerm, is usually richer in all the vitamins present than the original grain because the vitamins tend to be concentrated in those parts removed. Although we like to think of wheatbran as an excellent source of dietary fibre we should remember that it is also a rich provider of most of the B vitamins and vitamin E. Wheatgerm also is a highly significant source of these vitamins particularly in respect of vitamins B1 and E. Taken in isolation, all types of bran and cereal germs are very rich in the B vitamins (but not B12) and in vitamin E. For this reason they should be regarded, and indeed are by many people, as food supplements that can be added to other foods to enhance their vitamin levels.

Cooked items of cereal-based foods such as bread, cakes, biscuits, buns, pastries and puddings will also provide useful intakes of the vitamins present in the original cereals but will of necessity be at lower levels because of the cooking processes used. The addition of water and sugar, which do not provide vitamins to cooked cereal products will also dilute somewhat the vitamin content of the original cereals. White sugar supplies 'empty' calories, which means energy without the accompanying vitamins and minerals; brown and raw sugar do however contain some vitamins, as indeed does honey, but their contribution is not significant.

Milk and milk products

Milk has been described as the complete food since it contains all the main dietary constituents carbohydrate, fat and protein, plus a full spectrum of all the necessary vitamins and minerals needed for health. All it lacks is dietary fibre. This applies to whole milk but this can be subdivided into a fatty and an aqueous phase. Not surprisingly, therefore, the fatty or creamy part is rich in the fat soluble vitamins A, D and E and in the provitamin beta-carotene. Skimmed milk which comprises the main aqueous part of liquid milk, is therefore much richer in the water-soluble B vitamins complex and vitamin C and is virtually devoid of the fat-soluble vitamins. As butter is a concentrated form of milk fat it is an excellent source of all the fat-soluble vitamins (although, of course, butter, cream and full-cream milk are high in animal fats which raise the level of cholesterol in the blood); by a similar token dried skimmed milk supplies excellent quantities of all the B vitamins and vitamin C because they are concentrated by the removal of water. Similarly, cheese and yoghurt, produced from milk, retain the vitamin contents of the starting material. Indeed, since both are fermentation products it is possible for them, particularly yoghurt, to contain more B vitamins because of synthesis during the fermentative process. Milk, cheese and yoghurt are the sole significant sources of vitamin B12 in the diet of lactovegetarians who should ensure that these foods feature as part of their diet.

The practice of adding milk or cream to our cereals and mueslis therefore has some logic in providing a combination food that supplies a useful balance of all the vitamins needed in the diet. With the present-day trend of replacing whole milk by the skimmed variety to cut down dairy fat intake, to prevent the build-up of a high level of cholesterol related to heart disease, a valuable source of fat-soluble vitamins has been lost. It is essential, therefore, to make up this deficit by seeking out other foods to supply these essential fatty micronutrients.

Fats and oils
These food constituents can be disregarded as sources of all the B vitamins and vitamin C. They are, however, significant providers of the fat-soluble vitamins. In fact vegetable oils represent our most important dietary source of vitamin E. Not all vegetable oils contain the vitamin, for example, olive and coconut oils are virtually free of it, and this probably reflects the fact that these oils do not contain very much polyunsaturated fatty acids. It is a fact of nature that in general the higher

the content of these essential fatty acids in an oil, the higher is the vitamin E content. The vitamin functions in the seed or nut that contain these oils as a protecting agent of the polyunsaturated fatty acids. Similarly, cod liver oil, which is a rich source of these acids, is also high in vitamin E content.

In the absence of vitamin E, these polyunsaturated oils soon become rancid. Unfortunately, the processing required to extract these dietary oils like maize (corn), sunflower, safflower and soya, from the appropriate seed or grain will destroy or remove the vitamin E. Once the protective vitamin is removed and if it is not replaced, the oils break down rapidly when used in cooking processes and the resulting products can be quite toxic. Ensure, therefore, that the vegetable oil you buy contains vitamin E – if the vitamin is mentioned on the label you may assume it has been added and is perfectly acceptable.

Fats that have been produced from animal or fish sources contain vitamins A, D and E, although compound cooking fat and lard are virtually free of them because they have been processed out. The richest source of vitamins A and D are the fish liver oils but they can hardly be regarded as frequent or regular constituents of the diet. These oils can instead be taken in capsule form or by the teaspoonful as supplementary vitamins A and D.

Vitamin A as such does not actually occur in plant foods. However, vegetarians and vegans (extreme vegetarians) can obtain adequate intakes by means of the carotene which is in plants as the body is able to convert this into the vitamin as needed. Similarly, vitamin D does not occur in the commonly eaten plant foods. Despite the wide occurrence of carotene in plant foods, vegetable oils used in cooking or eaten raw on salads, contain only traces. The exception is unrefined palm oil, which is an extremely rich source of carotene, but this oil is hardly a common item of diet. The lack of vitamins A, D and carotene in edible vegetable oils means that when these are hardened and hence converted into margarine the resulting fat is devoid of these vitamins. For this reason, legislation now demands that all margarines are fortified with vitamin A or carotene and vitamin D to bring their levels up to those of butter. Vitamin E is readily destroyed by the hardening process that converts vegetable oils to margarines and often this vitamin too is added to these fats, although present legislation does not demand it. You should look for vitamin E, printed on the label and ensure that your brand contains it.

Meat and meat products

Muscle meats and products made from them are poor providers of vitamins A, D and carotene. They all contain some vitamin E but the concentrations are way below those found in vegetable oils. Most offal too is a poor source of vitamin A and carotene, but the vitamin E levels are somewhat higher than those in muscle meats. The exceptions are liver and kidney which provide very large amounts of vitamin A combined with significant intakes of vitamin D. Vitamin B levels are no higher than offal. Carotene contents vary amongst the livers from species and usually reflect the diet of the animal.

All muscle meats contain the whole spectrum of the water-soluble vitamin B complex but there is no vitamin C present at all. Again we must look to offal, particularly the liver and kidney, for the really rich providers of the vitamins – this time the B complex. Unlike muscle meats, all offal supplies useful quantities of vitamin C in the raw state but these tend to be reduced somewhat during cooking processes.

One of the most important B vitamins that we get from meat products is vitamin B12. These foodstuffs represent our most significant source of the vitamin and if these are not eaten as part of the diet, the chances of deficiency are increased. Lactovegetarians at least obtain their needs from dairy products (including eggs) but vegans should look to supplementation with the vitamin to ensure they are not deficient. Fortunately, unlike most B vitamins, substantial quantities of vitamin B12 are stored within the liver. The daily needs are so low (in the nature of one millionth of one gram) that once liver levels are built up, there is ample present for some time. The best way to accumulate vitamin B12 rapidly is to have it injected directly into the muscle but as this is the medical rather than the dietary approach, it is beyond the scope of readers of this book. Nevertheless, many vegans choose this method of taking their vitamin B12 in preference to a daily oral intake because injections are infrequent. Nevertheless, injection of the vitamin is the only solution if you are unable to absorb the vitamin from the diet. This condition, however, requires professional diagnosis and treatment.

Poultry and game

Apart from vitamin C which is not present in any poultry and game foods, all the vitamins are provided in significant quantities by these foodstuffs. The concentrations are similar to those of meats derived from animals.

Fish and seafoods

As eaten, white fish like cod, haddock, sole, plaice, halibut and whiting provide trace quantities only of vitamins A, D and of carotene. Some vitamin E is present but levels are rarely above one milligram per 100g (3.5oz). The only significant vitamins provided are those of the B complex and particularly vitamin B12. The quantity of vitamin C present in all these species is negligible. White fish should therefore be regarded primarily as good providers of the B vitamins only.

Fatty fish are different. Hence eels, herrings, bloaters, kippers, mackerel, pilchards, salmon, sardines, sprats, trout, tuna and whitebait are all useful suppliers of vitamins A, D and E but contain only traces of carotene. All the B vitamins are provided by these fish, at levels comparable to those in white wish, apart from vitamin B12 which occurs at much higher concentrations in fatty fish. Hence, apart from vitamin C, which is present in negligible quantities, the fatty fish provide the whole spectrum of vitamins in significant amounts. In this respect they are superior to white fish.

Cartilaginous fish, like dogfish and skate, provide few vitamins apart from members of the B complex and vitamin E.

Despite the fact that they are often regarded as delicacies, crustacea such as crab, lobster, prawns and shrimps provide little in the way of vitamins. Their main attributes are the presence of the vitamin B complex and of vitamin E, but levels are low relative to those fish and of meats. Molluscs like cockles, mussels, scallops and whelks too are not very rich providers of the vitamin B complex but do contain useful quantities of vitamin E. The only exception is oysters which supply significant quantities of vitamin A and higher levels of the vitamin B complex than do other molluscs.

Vegetables

All vegetables provide the whole range of B vitamins apart from B12 and.

although the concentrations are low, the relatively large amounts of vegetables eaten in the normal diet mean that they are an important source of these vitamins. Some high concentrations are however found in butter beans, haricot beans, mung beans, lentils, peas and potatoes, all of which are relatively rich in thiamine, riboflavin, nicotinic acid and pyridoxine, and the green-leafed vegetables are important providers of folic acid. Vegetarians are less likely than meat-eaters to be deficient in this B vitamin because of their high intake of leaf vegetables.

No vegetables contain vitamin A but all will provide carotene, the orange colouring agent which the body is able to convert into vitamin A. Even green vegetables contain carotene but its colour is masked by the stronger – coloured green chlorophyll. Hence green beans, brussels sprouts, broccoli, cabbage, lettuce, peas, spinach, spring greens, turnip tops, asparagus and watercress all are rich sources of carotene. When chlorophyll is absent, as in carrots, corn, sweet potatoes and tomatoes, the natural orange or yellow colour of carotene becomes more obvious and all are excellent providers of the vitamin A precursor. Vitamin D is however absent in vegetables. Most contain some vitamin E and, in view of the large amounts of vegetables eaten in the usual diet, significant quantities of the vitamin are obtained from these foodstuffs.

There is considerable variation in vitamin C contents amongst the vegetables but, as a general rule, the green-leafed varieties are richer than the beans, peas and root vegetables. The contribution of all vegetables in a good, mixed diet to our vitamin C intake is however significant. Potatoes are not a particularly rich source, especially when they are old, but in the Western world where they represent a staple part of the diet the sheer bulk eaten provides our main source of the vitamin. As most slimming regimes tend to avoid potatoes it is important to ensure other sources of vitamin C like vegetables and fruits are eaten to compensate for its lack in those undergoing such diets. New potatoes as picked are good providers of vitamin C but 80 percent can be lost as they age. Raw green peppers represent the richest vegetable source of vitamin C.

Fruits

Like vegetables, fruits do not contain any · vitamin A, but this is compensated by wide-ranging contents of the vitamin precursor carotene. Similarly fruits, like vegetables, do not contain any vitamin B12 or vitamin D, but there are unconfirmed reports that the latter vitamin is present in avocado pears. The rest of the B complex vitamins are present in all fruits, albeit at fairly low concentrations. Fruits also supply small amounts of vitamin E which, whilst useful as part of a varied diet, do not represent a particularly significant source when taken alone.

Although we tend to regard fruits as excellent sources of vitamin C, its concentration varies over a wide range in the various species. Pride of place goes to blackcurrants, gooseberries, oranges, grapefruit, lemons and limes, with pineapples also good providers of the vitamin. Unfortunately, the vitamin does not survive the drying process in the production of dried fruits which are virtually devoid of it. Apples provide varying quantities depending upon the variety – Sturmer Pippin represents the richest source, with Cox's at the other end of the scale.

Nuts

All nuts may be regarded as good sources of the B vitamins, with the exception of vitamin B12. They also feature as the richest sources of vitamin E amongst all foodstuffs. They are however completely lacking in vitamins A, D and carotene, and vitamin C levels are so low as to be disregarded. Roasted nuts however do tend to have lower levels of the B vitamins because of losses induced during the roasting process.

Other foods

Sugar, confectionery, jams, fruit spreads, marmalades, honey and preserves all provide only negligible quantities of the B vitamins and carotene or none at all. Jams and preserves contain some vitamin C provided by the fruit content but concentrations are not high. Chocolate products do provide reasonable amounts of the B vitamins, and vitamin E mainly by virtue of their cocoa and vegetable fat contents.

Beverages contain traces only of the B vitamins (apart from vitamin B12) with the exception of coffee which is a rich source of nicotinic acid. Instant coffee can contain as much as 39mg of this vitamin per 100g (3.5oz). Similarly, fruit juices provide only trace amounts of the B vitamins but their content of vitamin C is high enough to represent an important source of this vitamin.

Beers, lagers and wines all provide a wide spectrum of the B vitamins produced mainly during the fermentation process. Spirits, however, are completely devoid of all vitamins.

Soups will add some vitamins to the daily diet but the amounts present depend very much on the ingredients. Vegetables, meats and fowl that provide vitamins in their original state will also contribute them to the soup but the amount of processing the soup has been through will determine how many survive. When prepared from dried powders, the resulting soup is usually less nutritious in terms of its vitamin content than one of the tinned variety or, better still, one made from fresh ingredients.

Yeast is regarded as a good source of the B vitamins (apart from vitamin B12) particularly when it is dried. However, although a useful supplement, when taken in tablet form or sprinkled on food, dried yeast should not be regarded as a sole source of B vitamins since 100g (3.5oz) would have to be eaten daily to provide requirements. Most people could not tolerate the strong taste of this amount and at this level yeast could induce gout in susceptible people. Yeast should therefore be regarded simply as a useful vitamin B supplement when taken at the recommended dose.

Similarly, yeast extracts, which are concentrated from dried yeast, are extremely rich sources of the B vitamins (apart from vitamin B12, unless this is added) but they tend to be eaten in small amounts. Nevertheless, even at this level, they are very useful vitamin B supplements. Beef extracts will also provide excellent intakes of the B vitamins with the added advantage that they contain much more vitamin B12 than yeast extracts.

Non-dietary source of vitamins

Usually we tend to regard the diet as the main source of our vitamin needs under normal circumstances but some of them are supplied from non-dietary sources. Nicotinic acid, for example, can be made within body cells, particularly the liver, from the essential amino acid l-tryptophane. Although we define a vitamin as being an essential micronutrient that can be supplied only in the food, nicotinic acid is the exception. It is extremely doubtful that our complete requirements of nicotinic acid could be met by body synthesis from l-tryptophane because the rate of conversion is very inefficient. It has been calculated that it requires 60mg l-tryptophane to produce just 1 mg of nicotinic acid. Nevertheless this source can become significant when the vitamin is not being supplied directly in sufficient quantity by the diet. It must be said however that a diet poor in nicotinic acid is also likely to be poor also in good quality protein which supplies our dietary needs of l-tryptophane. Remember too that this amino acid has many other functions within the body, not only as a building block of tissue protein but as a precursor of brain substances needed for normal brain and nerve function. Its function as a precursor that can be converted to nicotinic acid must be regarded as minor but one that can assume importance when other sources of the vitamin are lacking. Good quality protein (e.g. from eggs, milk, meats, poultry, pulses, grains and seeds) will supply plenty of l-tryptophane enough to provide a useful supplementary supply of the vitamin.

Vitamin D is also synthesised within the body tissues by the action of sunlight upon the skin. Indeed this can supply such a proportion of the body's needs that it has been suggested that vitamin D should not be regarded as a vitamin at all! Whilst this may be true in those fortunate enough to live in a sunny climate all year round, many of those of us who do not will still require dietary sources of the vitamin. In fact one of the reasons why the vitamin D deficiency disease rickets appear in epidemic proportions in the industrial area of the UK and the rest of Europe was that the polluted air prevented the sunlight from falling on the skin of those living in these areas. When this factor was coupled with a poor intake of foods rich in the vitamin, perhaps it is not surprising deficiency developed.

The moral here is obvious. If you live in a cool climate ensure that whenever possible you get out into the sunshine so your body can make its own vitamin D. This vitamin is fat-soluble which means that it can be stored within the liver and fatty tissues of the body. The importance of this storage of vitamin D from the vitamin produced by the action of sunlight on the skin was demonstrated recently in a study of children from the East End of London. Half the children from one particular school were given two weeks' holiday at the seaside during the summer months. The other half stayed at home. All the children received a similar diet with virtually identical intakes of vitamin D from their food throughout the year. Six months after their summer holiday, those children who had spent just two weeks at the seaside had significantly higher levels of blood vitamin D than those who had stayed at home. A good insurance policy, then, is to build up your vitamin D supplies during the sunny weather by exposing the skin to the sun to stand you in good stead in the winter months when sunshine is less apparent. (Too much sunbathing is, of course, bad for the skin and can cause sunburn and even skin cancer). Look also to your dietary intakes during the winter, making sure your diet contains vitamin D-rich foods and even supplementing your diet with fish-liver-oils.

At the lower end of the large intestine there is a thriving population of bacteria which helps in the digestive and elimination processes. In fact about half of normal faeces consists of these bacteria which are eliminated along with waste good products. The bacteria, which are harmless, are usually nicely balanced to prevent over-production of the harmful bacteria and of the yeasts which can cause disease if allowed to flourish. Thrush is a good example of an infection due to yeasts which have been allowed to overproduce when the controlling effect of the 'friendly bacteria' has been lost. Lactobacilli represent one of the more important 'friendly bacteria' and as these are supplied in ample quantity by a living yoghurt the advantages of this food are obvious.

The introduction of powerful antibiotics to treat infective disease has however been shown to affect adversely the population of friendly bacteria that live in the large intestine. In addition to the pathogenic (harmful) bacteria that are destroyed by these antibiotics, the intestinal bacteria are also killed off, with the result that some vitamins normally synthesized by them are no longer available to the body. This is because such bacteria have the ability to make vitamins for their own use which can later be absorbed and utilized by the body. Amongst the vitamins known to be produced by the intestinal bacteria are biotin, pantothenic acid and vitamin K. We know this because studies have indicated that people can excrete more of these vitamins than was present in the food eaten. The excess must therefore have been supplied within the intestinal tract. Also it is known that long-term antibiotic treatment can give rise to deficiencies of biotin and of vitamin K because these vitamins are no longer being supplied by the intestinal bacteria. When dietary intakes of these vitamins are low, their synthesis by the 'friendly bacteria' then assumes great importance. It is likely that all the vitamins are made to some extent by the 'friendly bacteria' but most of them, with the exception of those mentioned previously, are either produced in such low potency as to be of little help to the host or they are produced too far down the intestinal tract to be absorbed.

Recent studies though have indicated that in some people, the intestinal bacteria can provide significant quantities of vitamin B12 that can be absorbed and made available to the host. Usually the vitamin cannot be assimilated because when produced in this way it is too far down the intestine to be absorbed. Some people, however, for one reason or another have bacterial populations that live much higher up in the intestinal tract than is usual – so high in fact that the vitamin B12 produced can be utilized. Such people are those who live in areas of the world where the standard of hygiene is lower perhaps than that desired by more fortunate populations, in other words the inhabitants of most Third World countries. This goes a long way in explaining why such individuals, whilst lacking the B12-rich foods like meats and dairy products in their diets nevertheless do not develop vitamin B12 deficiency. Similarly, it now looks as if vegans and other extreme vegetarians may, because of their diet, develop bacterial populations higher up the intestine than meat-eaters and so benefit from locally-produced vitamin B12. However, vegans in particular would be well advised to take a supplementary form of vitamin B12 daily. This is because bacterial synthesis may produce just enough of the vitamin to prevent the symptoms of deficiency but it may not suffice to provide the quantity required for optimum health.

The best example of complete synthesis of vitamin needs within the body is provided by ruminants like cattle, sheep and goats. These animals possess a rumen, one of their four stomachs, that acts like a fermentation tank. Within this, the bacterial population produces all the members of the vitamin B complex from nutrients supplied in the forage. Although some of these vitamins are introduced in the diet, significant quantities are produced within the rumen. Vitamin B12 is synthesized in large quantities by this natural process so these animals are highly unlikely to suffer a deficiency even though the vitamin is not supplied in their vegetarian diet. The only time that ruminants may be prone to vitamin B12 deficiency is when the soil on which they graze, and hence the food that they eat, is deficient in the mineral cobalt. When this is lacking, the rumen bacteria cannot synthesize vitamin B12.

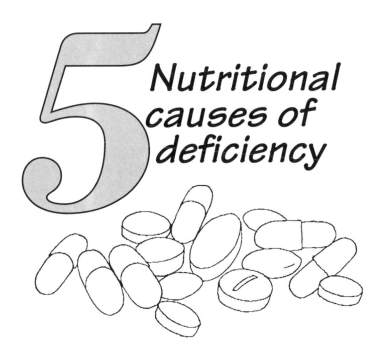

5 Nutritional causes of deficiency

Poor storage of food, cooking methods that do not retain the full vitamin potency of food items and inefficient utilization of cooking fluids can all cause significant losses of vitamins. In addition there are many other factors that can give rise to vitamin deficiency and most individuals will be prone to the influence of one or more. Let us now consider these so that if you can identify them as being relevant to yourself you will be able to take steps to remedy any potential deficiency.

Apathy

This is often a feature of people living alone, within all age groups, but particularly in those who have lost a spouse and perhaps no longer have a family to look after. There is little incentive to prepare adequate meals which are often monotonous and not nourishing enough. Impaired digestive ability may be associated with the apathy and this may exacerbate the low nutritional status of the individual. The apathetic approach to eating is often seen in the elderly middle-aged bachelor or spinster living in accommodation with poor cooking facilities, or in teenagers and students who are living alone for the first time. The obvious remedy is to pay more attention to the diet in conjunction perhaps with an all-round multivitamin supplement.

Dental problems

Poor dentition, for whatever reason, whether loss of teeth, dental decay or ill-fitting dentures, can make eating uncomfortable. The result is an aversion to foods that require a lot of chewing, such as salads, meats and vegetables. As these food items are important suppliers of the whole range of vitamins needed, the chances of deficiency developing are increased when they are not provided in the diet. A filling, though ill-balanced diet, must inevitably lead to a mild deficiency of vitamins. Poor dental health will contribute to it, so improving this must be the first step in ensuring a well-balanced and hence healthier diet.

Food fads

Nutritional imbalances are often seen when excessive quantities of particular items of food, usually of the 'empty-calorie' variety, are eaten at the expense of other more nutritionally desirable foodstuffs. Young people are particularly prone to this factor of imbalance when they prefer high calorie but low vitamin content foods, such as sugar-rich foods, soft drinks, confectionery, potato snacks, sweets, cakes and the like, to more basic but less attractive (at least to them) foods. Old people are not immune to food fad diets either and will often partake of excessive intakes of beverages, processed cereals and preserves to the detriment of more nourishing foods. The food fads sometimes associated with pregnancy do not have the same significance because they are variable and usually of a temporary nature. It has been suggested that they may be satisfying a demand by the woman for specific nutrients and so should not be discouraged. Other food fads should, however, be regarded as contributing to an insidious development of mild vitamin deficiencies and should be treated by improving the diet or, failing this, by at least ensuring the minimum daily requirements of these micronutrients with a good multivitamin preparation.

Food taboos

They tend to arise because of religious beliefs but these, in turn, are often a logical response to knowledge about the food based on bitter experience. Meat that is prone to parasitic infection is often avoided for obvious reason but there can be unwanted results. For example, when pork is taboo, the richest meat source of thiamine is denied and the chances of developing a mild deficiency are increased accordingly. Dairy products based on cow's milk are often avoided avidly by some people but in so doing they are depriving themselves of a rich source of vitamin D and the B complex vitamin B2. Unless other food sources of these are eaten, a mild deficiency will develop. Some people, of course, are genuinely afraid of products based on cow's milk because of allergic reactions to them so they must look to other ways of obtaining these vitamins.

Those who do not eat meat or poultry products (or even fish) like vegetarians and those who are even more extreme like those who avoid all food products of animal origin may also be regarded as food faddists. Their main concern should be their intake of dietary vitamin B12 which is available to really significant amounts only from foods of animal origin. They should be aware that vitamin B12 deficiency, and, in the case of vegans, riboflavin deficiency is far more likely because of their dietary habits. The supplementary vitamin, made by fermentation and hence of non-animal source, is essential for them to receive optimal intakes.

In some cases of food taboos, specific foods that are nutritionally sound are avoided because of an unfounded belief that they do harm. Many such beliefs abound in Africa, South America and the Far East. In Bolivia, for example, any food containing animal blood is believed to make children mute so it is avoided during pregnancy by the mother and withheld from the child after birth. In West Pakistan, buffalo milk is quite erroneously believed to produce great physical strength but to reduce the mental ability of the person who drinks it. Hence a nutritious food is avoided by many – a situation made even more tragic when this food represents a potentially important source of protein, vitamins and minerals. Unfortunately, in these parts of the world many food taboos are confined to the pregnant woman who is thus often deprived of the very nutrients she desperately requires.

Fasting

Complete avoidance of food or fasting is often a feature of many religious sects. The occasional 24-hour fast, believed by some to be a useful practice in purging the body of toxins and poisons, probably does little harm in terms of reducing vitamin intakes. Where extensive fasting is undertaken as in Ramadan, however, there is almost certainly nutritional harm done. Whether this affects the health and eventual life span of Moslem people has not been studied, but logic would suggest that the lack of vitamins and minerals taken in over long periods must deplete their levels in the body. Water-soluble vitamins, because they are not stored to any great extent, are the most likely to be depleted during prolonged fasting. Fat soluble vitamins are stored in the liver and fatty tissues of the body so during periods of normal eating, sufficient of these are retained to supply requirements when food intake is stopped.

Individual requirements

These are usually expressed by official bodies as recommended dietary intakes or as recommended daily allowances. They are regarded as sufficient to prevent symptoms of deficiency diseases but not necessarily sufficient to maintain optimum health. Three criteria are used to assess these levels:

1. They take account of individual variations in requirements by introducing a safety factor to cover 95 percent of the population.

2. They take account of possible increase caused by the minor stresses of life but extra needs during infection, injuries and other illnesses are ignored.

3. They are unlikely to take account of different availability of vitamins in various foods.

Despite these assurances, the wide range of suggested daily intakes amongst various countries with similar ethnic groups would suggest that none of them are really aware of what our needs are. Why, for example, do the Russians and Rumanians regard 75 to 85mg vitamin C as a desirable daily intake, while in the United Kingdom only 30mg is regarded as adequate? Similarly, these Eastern Bloc countries suggest that vitamin A needs for their people are twice those that the Department of Health in the UK regarded as sufficient for Britons. Fortunately, the EC recommendations coming into force are more realistic intakes.

Experiments indicate that animals of the same species can vary one from another in their vitamin requirements by anything from two to ten-fold. Often, although the lower figures represents what is needed to prevent abject signs of deficiency, the higher figure is that required for optimum health. A similar situation applies also to human beings. Two people on a similar diet can show wide variation in their blood levels of vitamins, suggesting that individual human needs are also different. Hence the individual with the higher requirements can be suffering from a mild deficiency of some vitamins simply because his requirements are not met from a diet that would supply adequate intakes for someone else. Without extensive testing no one can determine their exact requirements with any accuracy but if benefit is felt from an all-round vitamin supplement taken regularly, it would suggest that their needs are not met by the diet.

To illustrate varying official views on what their people need in the way of daily vitamin intakes, the following figures are taken from American, UK, USSR and EC authorities respectively:

OFFICIAL RECOMMENDED DAILY VITAMIN INTAKES			
	USA	*UK*	*USSR*	*EC*
VITAMIN A (μg)	750	1,000	1,500	800
VITAMIN D (μg)	7.0	2.5	10	5.0
VITAMIN E (mg)	15	–	–	10
THIAMIN (mg)	1.4	1.1	1.8	1.4
RIBOFLAVIN (mg)	1.6	1.7	2.4	1.6
NICOTINIC ACID (mg)	20	19	25	18
PANTOTHENIC ACID(mg)	7.0	–	10.0	6.0
PYRIDOXINE (mg)	2.0	–	2.1	2.0
BIOTIN (mg)	100	–	–	150
FOLIC ACID (μg)	400	300	500	200
VITAMIN B12 (μg)	3.5	2.0	5.0	1.0
VITAMIN C (mg)	45	30	80	60

N.B. Blanks indicate that no particular level is recommended.

These figures should be regarded merely as a guideline. There is no reason why with a good diet they not be doubled at least. The higher the intake the more likely it is that requirements for optimum health are achieved, at least up to certain limits. When the diet cannot supply such needs, supplementation then becomes essential.

Other food nutrients

The need for vitamins may be increased by other food constituents. Vitamin levels may also be reduced under the influence of other nutrients. Prime examples of these factors are seen with high polyunsaturated fats intakes, a trend that is increasing amongst the health-conscious public. Unless the requisite vitamin E is taken at the same time, high levels of these fats can induce deficiency of the vitamin. In fact, the simplest way to make experimental animals vitamin E deficient in order to study the effects, is to feed large amounts of polyunsaturated vegetable oils that are devoid of the vitamin. Not only is their vitamin E intake decreased but the body levels of the vitamin are drastically reduced.

Any increase in dietary calories, especially of the empty kind, will need a concomitant rise in thiamine intake as the two are related. When the vitamin in the diet does not keep pace with these empty calories, a mild deficiency will gradually develop. This is probably one of the main causes of the widespread increase in mild thiamine deficiency that is being observed today in the Western world.

In a similar manner, high dietary intakes of protein should be accompanied by increased vitamin B6 in the diet. Fortunately, high protein foods tend to contain high B6 levels, but if these are destroyed by poor cooking techniques or other destructive factors, an imbalance will occur. Alternatively, when protein intakes are low, less vitamin B6 is required.

Specific amino acids in the diet (as part of the food protein) can also influence vitamin levels. We have seen that low tryptophane levels in the diet can reduce nicotinic acid concentrations because the amino acids act as a precursor of the vitamin. At the same time, another amino acid, leucine, when present in high-dietary concentrations needs extra nicotinic acid. A food high in leucine and low in tryptophane, such as millet, is therefore conducive to nicotinic acid deficiency. Hence, in those countries where millet is the staple diet, the chances of this particular deficiency are increased.

Some proteins can cause inactivation or destruction of vitamins. Avidin is a protein unique to raw egg-white that combines with and inactivates the B-vitamin biotin. When the egg-white is cooked, avidin is destroyed so the full potency of the vitamin is available. The moral is to avoid high intakes of raw egg-white.

Another food that can cause destruction of vitamins is raw fish. The reason is that this foodstuff contains an enzyme called thiaminase which specifically destroys thiamine. Thiaminase, like all enzymes, is protein in nature so it is destroyed when the food containing it is cooked. In some parts of the world, notably the Far East, raw fish is a staple part of the diet so the chances of this inducing a thiamine deficiency are increased. At the same time thiamine can be easily inactivated by a bacterium called Bacillus thiaminolyticus which is a common infective micro-organism of raw fish. A combination of these two factors in the diet of Japanese is believed to be the reason why three percent of the population suffer mild deficiency of thiamine. In the West where we tend to cook our fish before eating it, the problems do not arise because both the thiaminase and the microorganism are destroyed by the cooking process.

Other vitamins

Excessive intakes of one vitamin may induce deficiency of another. Such situations may not arise very often in everyday life but it has been established that very high intakes of folic acid can cause a deficiency of vitamin B12. This can happen in vegetarians and in particular vegans, who combine high dietary levels of folic acid (present in vegetables) with much reduced intakes of vitamin B12 (present in fish, animal foods and dairy products). An imbalance of folic acid and vitamin B12 intakes in the daily diet can also lead to clinical complications. If a vegetarian or vegan loses the ability to absorb vitamin B12, their high folic acid intake will mask the anaemia caused by deficiency of the B12. What is not masked is the insidious degeneration of the spinal cord that is an additional feature of vitamin B12 deficiency. A stage is eventually reached when the nervous system is damaged beyond repair. It is therefore important that vitamin B12 deficiency is diagnosed rapidly in vegans and vegetarians and this is the province of the medical practitioner. For this reason, too, the availability of the vitamin B12 and folic acid in products on sale to the public is confined to those containing only a low potency. This is to avoid overdosage with folic acid masking a possible deficiency of vitamin B12.

Other vitamin interactions that have been observed are high levels of carotene inducing a vitamin D deficiency when vitamin D intakes are on the borderline. When vitamin C is missing, folic acid deficiency symptoms can manifest themselves. This is because vitamin C is essential for the folic acid in the body to be converted to its metabolic active form, folinic acid. Even if folic acid is present at high concentration it is useless unless there is sufficient vitamin C available to activate it. Both vitamins must therefore be present for folic acid-deficiency anaemia to be avoided.

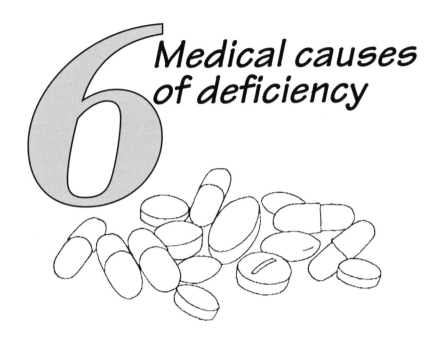

6 Medical causes of deficiency

Excessive losses from the body

As most of the vitamins are water-soluble they will tend to be eliminated in the watery excretion of the body such as sweat, tears and urine. When diarrhoea is present, the watery faeces may also contain excessive amounts of vitamins because, in this condition, absorption of vitamins is curtailed and hence more readily excreted. Losses through perspiration can be significant in excessive physical exertion, as in athletes, or as a result of living in hot climates. Tobacco smoke can inactivate vitamin C. Alcohol can cause excessive release of the B vitamins and vitamin C from the liver and hence from the body via the urine. Alcohol is also able to inhibit absorption of some vitamins from the food. These vitamin losses must be replaced by an improved diet or by supplementation with a multivitamin preparation.

Infections

Any sort of bacterial or viral infection can give rise to deficiencies of vitamins A and C. On the other hand, infections are more likely in those suffering from malnutrition and hence vitamin deficiency, particularly amongst children. Infections can aggravate malnutrition by reducing the appetite and, in turn, malnutrition weakens resistance to illness – a vicious circle indeed. The infections most likely to occur in malnourished children are bacterial (e.g. tuberculosis), viral (e.g. measles which can be a killing disease in malnutrition) and those due to parasites.

The ultimate result of vitamin A deficiency upon the eye is a condition called keratomalacia which induces blindness but is aggravated by any concurrent infections. Vitamin deficiency may lower resistance to infection by a reduced antibody formation; reduced activity of the white blood cells (phagocytes) which usually engulf invading bacteria and viruses; decrease the levels of protective enzymes (e.g. lysozyme, an enzyme in tears that protects the eyes); reduce the integrity of the skin and mucous membranes, the wet surfaces of the body, and so allowing invading micro-organisms to flourish. At one time vitamin A was referred to as 'the anti-infective vitamin' but now we know that all the vitamins, in one way or another, contribute to the body's resistance to disease. Adequate intakes of the whole range will therefore contribute to the defences of the body.

Infections can precipitate gross deficiencies of vitamins in those on a poor diet and even mild deficiencies in those on an adequate diet. For example, children with meningitis, diarrhoea, tuberculosis, measles and other acute infections can develop vitamin deficiency severe enough to cause them to develop keratomalacia and, eventually, blindness. Glandular fever (infective mono-nucleosis) is notorious in inducing deficiency across the range of vitamins and supplementation with a high potency multivitamin preparation should be taken by those with this infection, particularly during the period of convalescence. All types of fever can cause symptoms of scurvy in children due to vitamin C deficiency, even when there appear to be adequate dietary intakes. Thiamine deficiency caused by fever can drop to such levels as to give rise to the symptoms of beriberi, the ultimate deficiency disease.

Infections often cause loss of appetite, so vitamin intake is much reduced and this is exacerbated by losses due to the infection. Hence supplementation during the period of convalescence following the illness is most important since even a return to a normal appetite is unlikely to rapidly make up the deficit of vitamins caused in the first place by the infection.

Malabsorption syndromes

There are several clinical conditions which are characterised by an inability of the individual to absorb the micro nutrients in the diet. Most of these conditions result in fat malabsorption and since the fat soluble vitamins A, D, E and K are absorbed by the same mechanisms as dietary fats, they too are not absorbed or are absorbed only to a limited extent. Only one water-soluble vitamin B12, is affected by a malabsorption syndrome.

Impaired absorption of fats and fat soluble vitamins is a feature of the following diseases: sprue, idiopathic steatorrhoea, pancreatic disease, lack of bile production due to liver disease, gall bladder blockage and any disease affecting the production of fat-splitting digestive enzymes and bile salts. The latter are essential for emulsifying fats, a necessary prerequisite to their digestion and absorption.

Vitamin B12 may be present in adequate amounts in the diet but there are some conditions where it cannot be absorbed. The reason is that the vitamin is assimilated into the body by a unique mechanism. It must be complexed with a specific protein called intrinsic factor before absorption can take place. For some reason, certain people cease producing intrinsic factor and the resulting lack of B12 absorption gives rise to pernicious anaemia. Treatment of this condition can only be carried out successfully with intramuscular injections of the vitamin. It is, therefore, a matter of correct diagnosis of pernicious anaemia first, followed by medical treatment with injectable B12 and for these reasons therapy must be left to the medical practitioner.

Medicinal drugs

The common medicinal drugs, some of them available without prescription, may affect the nutritional status of the individual taking them. Some of these drugs increase the requirement for certain of the vitamins. For example, the synthetic oestrogens and progestogens in the contraceptive pill may increase the woman's need for vitamin B6.

She must, therefore, take extra vitamin B6 to satisfy her requirements and often the quantity of the vitamin in her diet, even if this is highly nutritious, is not sufficient. It is essential for her, therefore, to take a vitamin B6 supplement, usually between 25 and 100mg daily.

Drugs may also interfere with the absorption of some vitamins so that when the medicine is taken with food the full nutritional benefit of that food is not obtained. Folic acid and vitamin B12, for example, are poorly absorbed in the presence of para-aminosalicylic acid (used to treat tuberculosis); phenytoin (a drug used to treat epilepsy) and colchicine (used to treat gout). There are however two important exceptions to this. First, when taking phenytoin, folic acid supplements should not be taken without medical advice. This is because excess folic acid may neutralise the beneficial effect of the drug. Second, extra vitamin B6 should not be taken with the drug levodopa (used in Parkinson's disease) because the vitamin interferes with the beneficial action of the drug.

Some drugs may interfere with the utilisation and activation of vitamins. The best example of this is the medicine liquid paraffin which has been widely used to act as an intestinal lubricant in cases of constipation. Liquid paraffin dissolves the fat-soluble vitamins present in the diet or in supplements and prevents them being absorbed. As liquid paraffin is neither digested nor absorbed, the vitamins become trapped within it and are no longer available for absorption through the intestinal system. The occasional use of liquid paraffin as an anti-constipation agent has no significant effect upon the fat-soluble vitamins, but when taken constantly, for example by the aged, the liquid paraffin may immobilise the fat-soluble vitamins to such an extent that deficiency is possible. The treatment is to take the fat soluble vitamins as supplements at a different time of day to that when liquid paraffin is taken. Alternatively, in really severe cases, the vitamins can be injected in order to bypass the intestine and the problems with liquid paraffin. Another way to overcome the problem is to take the fat-soluble vitamins in a water-solubilised form so that they are then not available for solution into the liquid paraffin. Typical daily supplements are between 2,500 and 7,500 i.u. vitamin A; 200 to 400 i.u. vitamin D and up to 250 i.u. vitamin E. Vitamin K should be taken at the discretion of a medical practitioner.

Aspirin is one of the most widely used analgesic drugs yet its effect upon vitamin C has been known since 1936. When aspirin was taken by children, the urinary excretion of vitamin C increased. Two aspirin tablets (600mg of the active drug acetylsalicylic acid) taken by healthy adults every six hours were found to result in a 100 percent increase in the 24-hour excretion of ascorbic acid. An intake of aspirin such as this (2.4g or 8 aspirin tablets daily) is not unusual in the treatment of arthritic conditions, so anyone undertaking this therapy should be aware of a possible vitamin C deficiency.

A constant feature in arthritic patients is reduced levels of vitamin C in their white blood cells. As these cells act in the blood as scavengers of infective bacteria and viruses, and as their efficiency in this respect is dependent on adequate vitamin C levels, it is not surprising that many arthritis sufferers being treated with aspirin are prone to infections. Studies reported in *The Lancet* concluded that between 200 and 300mg of vitamin C should be swallowed with every two aspirin tablets.

There are other benefits to be gained from taking vitamin C with aspirin. Apart from simple replacement of the vitamin C lost, the vitamin also increases the efficacy of aspirin by increasing its absorption. This, in turn, leads to faster pain relief, a slower rate of excretion of the drug and longer duration of its action. The well-known side-effects of aspirin taken alone include gastric discomfort, blood loss, sedation and reduced vitamin C status. All of these reactions are reduced by taking extra vitamin C, but it must be eaten simultaneously with the drug. Studies reported in *The Lancet* in 1968 indicated that aspirin is more likely to cause gastric bleeding when vitamin C levels in the individual are low.

The conditions for which aspirin is taken, including the common cold, influenza, rheumatoid arthritis and osteoarthritis, themselves create a greater requirement for vitamin C. Treating such diseases with aspirin will therefore worsen the deficiency of the vitamin. Remember, too, that the ability of the body to fight off infections and to heal itself and reduce inflammation is very much dependent on a good supply of vitamin C. Aspirin may therefore be depleting the body of the very vitamin it needs for its own protection. Also remember that these effects of aspirin are shared to some extent by the non-steroidal anti-inflammatory drugs used to treat arthritis.

Corticosteroids (steroid drugs), used in medicine for a wide variety of diseases and conditions also induce excretion of vitamin C. In addition though, vitamin B6 is affected to such an extent that increased requirements are needed to maintain normal body levels. The mineral zinc is also excreted under the influence of corticosteroid drugs and this too should feature in the diet of those taking these drugs over prolonged periods. It is not without significance that anyone who is treated with corticosteroid drugs over any length of the time usually finds that any wounds they suffer will take a longer time to heal than in those who are not taking such drugs. We know that vitamin C and zinc are both essential to the healing of wounds so their excessive losses due to the steroid drugs may well be factors in determining a slow healing rate.

Administration of antibiotics, such as the tetracycline's, have been found to lower the level of vitamin C in the white blood cells and in the blood plasma. The reason is that the antibiotic appears to prevent the normal conservation of the vitamin by the kidneys so it is lost. The resulting white blood cell levels of vitamin C cause a reduced ability to resist infection. Hence patients, such as those with chronic bronchitis who are on prolonged regular treatment with antibiotics, are at risk of both an impaired vitamin C status and weakened natural defence mechanisms. The young should also be aware of this vitamin C-wasting effect of tetracycline antibiotics since low doses of them are often prescribed for very long periods in the treatment of acne. Vitamin C supplementation at levels up to 500mg daily becomes essential for anyone on long-term antibiotic treatment.

There is little doubt that antibiotics in general can have a deleterious effect upon the intestinal bacteria which under normal circumstances are useful providers of some of the B-vitamins and of vitamin K. Not only is the body deprived of these vitamins by the destruction caused by the antibiotics but replenishment of the friendly bacteria is curtailed as their normal balance is upset. Redressing the balance is best carried out by supplementing the diet with the B complex at fairly high potencies. At the same time, eating natural yoghurt is often recommended because it is a rich source of the friendly bacteria organisms. Taking the vitamin B complex with antibiotics and, indeed after the drug treatment has finished, will prevent the gastro-intestinal side-effects often associated with this type of therapy.

We have seen how various drugs most commonly used in medicine can upset the vitamin balance of the body. Replenishment with the vitamin is usually straightforward. There are, however, many other drugs that can affect vitamin status so extra vitamins are useful. Many treatments, of course, are short-term and perhaps in these cases any effect upon vitamins is transitory and so they tend to be ignored. You should be aware though of any prolonged medicinal therapy that can upset the nutritional basis of the body and protect yourself accordingly by taking the right supplements.

Parasitic infections

These include the various worm infections that can thrive in the intestinal tract. The worms utilise the vitamins in the diet before the micro nutrients can be absorbed, so a deficiency can be induced. The most likely vitamin to be affected is B12 because this is present in minute quantities anyway and parasitic worms have a particular affinity for this vitamin.

Poor digestion

This condition can be a contributory factor in causing certain vitamin deficiencies. Digestive upsets can arise because of defective chewing of food; by a reduction in the volume and acidity of gastric secretions; by inefficient production of digestive enzymes in the pancreatic, liver and intestinal juices; by a reduction in bile secretion, affecting mainly the fat-soluble vitamins. When a meal is eaten, the vitamins are liberated only as the food is digested. Hence a defective digestion system will not allow the vitamins to be presented for absorption at the right spot in the intestinal tract and a slow, insidious deficiency may develop.

Rapid growth

When a foetus is in the developing stage within the womb, all the vitamins are needed for its growth. These are supplied via the blood of the mother, so her dietary intakes of vitamins must satisfy her own needs as well as those of the developing baby. Once born, a child needs vitamins for its growth as well as for normal metabolism. Many animal studies have indicated that the offspring who do not have intakes of vitamins adequate for both purposes will suffer in their growth process. A similar situation applies also to the growing child whose vitamin intakes must be optimum rather than simply adequate. Most authorities agree that the need for vitamins in children is relatively higher than that in adults, when worked out on a body-weight or food-intake basis.

Population sectors that are likely to be vitamin deficient

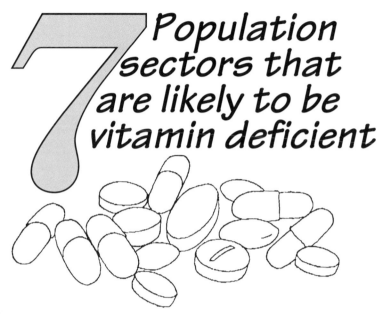

A vitamin deficiency can occur in two ways. In the first, a primary deficiency can be caused by an inadequate diet resulting in a reduced intake over a long period of time. This may be months or years in the case of those vitamins like A and B12 which are stored to a great extent during periods of adequate intakes. Most vitamins, however, have a high turnover which means that a deficiency manifests itself fairly quickly once intakes start to drop.

In the second way a conditioned deficiency arises out of an adequate diet where other factors affect the vitamin intake. These factors may decrease the absorption of vitamins; prevent their release from the food eaten; cause increased requirements over and above those in an adequate diet; increase their turnover; or give rise to enhanced excretion. In the previous section these factors were discussed but it is because they can induce deficiency that many authorities are now questioning the concept of an average vitamin intake from the diet. It is quite likely that each individual has his or her vitamin requirements peculiar to themselves. These can, of course, fall below those recommended as the norm but it is more likely they will be higher.

Hence it is now recognised that not only individuals can vary in their vitamin requirements but there do exist various sectors in the population who by their very nature are likely to need more vitamins to maintain health. Although these extra vitamin needs could, in theory, be met by improving the diet, in many cases this is not always possible or practicable, so supplementary sources must be sought. In addition, some people's need for vitamins is so high that there is no way these levels can be obtained even from a very good diet.

Many nutritional studies have indicated which sectors of the population are likely to require vitamins and these will now be discussed. If you find you fit into one of these population sectors, the chances are that you should be looking to your vitamin intake. The benefits obtained by a diet change or simple supplementation will outweigh any nominal cost involved.

Are you elderly?

Various studies on vitamins in the elderly have drawn attention to many aspects of nutrition in those of advancing years. No one is quite sure of their vitamin requirements, nor do they know to what extent these vitamins are absorbed from the food eaten. It is highly likely that the efficiency of absorption decreases as a person ages, so naturally more must be eaten. This was demonstrated quite clearly in one study where old people living in an institution were eating an adequate diet with ample vitamin levels yet their body content was invariably low. Only by a general vitamin supplementation were body levels of vitamins restored to where they should have been. One note of interest was the immediate benefit to health experienced.

Other factors contributing to a decreased intake of micronutrients in old people include a host of social, psychological and economic influences. Some more specific problems in this area are poor dentition leading to an aversion to vitamin-rich foods like salads, whole grains and meat; a reluctance for physical or emotional reasons to shop frequently for a wide variety of foodstuffs; loss of a spouse leading to a reluctance to cook food, with undue reliance on refined carbohydrates and beverages of doubtful nutritional value; excessive losses of vitamin due to the methods used in mass cooking of meals where these form the staple diet. All these factors can reduce vitamin intake.

Vitamin malnutrition may lead to a much worse state of affairs resulting in a phase of sub-clinical nutrition which can lead to poor health, apathy and disinterest – a vicious circle too common in elderly people. The most common deficiencies encountered were those of vitamin B1 (thiamine), vitamin C and vitamins A and D. The problem has reached such a level that the writer of a leading article in the *British Medical Journal* feels it would be beneficial to offer people of an advanced age supplements like liquid milk fortified with vitamin D. This would be a useful source of vitamins and minerals as well as the milk protein and calories which older people may also lack.

It would also be beneficial to any old person to be given iron, vitamin B complex, vitamin C and the fat-soluble vitamins A and D for some weeks following an illness or operation. Vitamins are needed for overcoming the effects of illness and for the rapid healing of wounded tissue and any lack of these nutrients to the aged must have a deleterious effect upon recovery.

A report of the Panel on Nutrition of the Elderly drew attention to the fact that the lack of sunlight falling onto the skin of housebound old people would predispose them to a deficiency of vitamin D, leading to softening of the bones, a disease called osteomalacia. This condition, the adult counterpart of childhood rickets, may also be complicated by osteoporosis – a literal honeycombing of the bone leading to easy breakage. It now looks like an adequate intake of vitamin D and calcium throughout life will reduce considerably the chances of developing these conditions in old age. Vitamin D is best taken to prevent the development of osteomalacia and osteoporosis, which you can do on a self-help basis rather than wait for the diseases to appear and then be treated professionally.

Many studies indicate that vitamin C intakes in the elderly are low and these are reflected in the findings that body levels in these people are also reduced. Although few overt signs of scurvy appear, these low levels probably contribute to the generalised malaise often observed in the elderly – a condition that usually responds to simple supplementation with vitamin C even at the moderate intake of 100mg daily.

Other investigators have reported that thiamine, riboflavin and nicotinic acid also tend to be reduced in both the intakes and the bodies of the elderly. As these three B vitamins comprise the so-called 'energy vitamins', then effects of their deficiency on the activity of older people can be imagined. Again, simple low-level supplementation with these vitamins can often change an old person's outlook on life considerably, leading to a whole new lifestyle. Vitamin B12 is also at risk, mainly because of reduced intakes of meat, poultry, fish and dairy products by the elderly.

Certain other factors make old people especially liable to mild malnutrition. They include limited mobility, loneliness and social isolation which in turn often lead to apathy, depression and impairment of appetite. The whole situation can become a vicious circle when applied particularly to the elderly disabled or to the housebound.

The obvious remedy for any ageing person is to improve the diet in terms of quality and by attempting to balance the intake of foodstuffs to ensure that all the vitamins are supplied. This, however, is easier said than done, and a simple all-round multivitamin preparation (sometimes with minerals) taken daily will at least ensure the minimum intake of vitamins without reference to those in the food. During the winter months, extra vitamin C (say 300 to 500mg daily) may also be needed to ward off infections that are prevalent at that time of the year.

Are you pregnant or breast-feeding?

It is well established that there are profound metabolic changes associated with pregnancy, some of which continue even after the mother has given birth and starts breast-feeding her child. During pregnancy the mother becomes more efficient in her utilization of both protein and energy, laying down considerable reserves during the first six months. These reserves are then drawn upon during the last three months and throughout the period when she is breast-feeding. Whilst protein and energy (in the form of fat) can be stored within the body, there is nowhere that the water-soluble vitamins can be accumulated for later use. Hence the fact that all authorities who recommend minimum daily intakes of vitamins suggest extra intakes during pregnancy and breast feeding.

The mother needs extra vitamins to ensure, first, the growth of the baby inside her and second, to supply the body, once born, with adequate vitamin reserves. The increased demand for vitamins increases whilst she is breast feeding because the suckling's needs are met only from the mother's milk. Obviously, if the mother is to meet those increased needs of nutrients (including vitamins) by eating ordinary foods then she will have to eat greater quantities. Once her needs and those of the child are reached, any excess calories will be laid down as fat and obesity may then become a problem.

The answer, to prevent excessive calorie intake whilst maintaining adequate vitamin levels, is thus to take extra of those micronutrients in the form of supplements. Many women are supplied with these by their medical practitioner but it is likely that all pregnant women will benefit from supplementation. This should be at a level sufficient to provide the extra requirements during pregnancy and breast feeding, and there is no point in taking more than is necessary. Although high intakes of vitamins have never been proved to be detrimental to the mother or to the foetus, apart perhaps from vitamin A, neither is it known with certainty if these intakes are safe. The UK authorities, for example, recommend no more than 2,250μg (7,500 i.u.) vitamin A to be taken daily as a supplement during pregnancy.

The safest regime is best worked out from the table overleaf which indicates what various authorities suggest to the pregnant and nursing mother. At least these will ensure that no one suffers even mild deficiency.

Many studies have indicated that pregnant women are most likely to suffer from marked decreases in their blood levels of vitamin A, nicotinic acid, pyridoxine, vitamin B12 and vitamin C. To these must now be added the B vitamin folic acid. Pyridoxine is one vitamin that has been studied with reference to its requirements during pregnancy.

The existence of a pyridoxine deficiency in pregnancy has been suspected for over 30 years but the medical profession has never agreed as to the value of giving the vitamin during this period of a woman's life. One study that attempted to resolve the problem was carried out in West Germany in 1973. Of the 458 women with uncomplicated pregnancies who were studied, between 40 and 60 percent were found to be low in vitamin B6 on all the criteria measured.

It can, therefore, be assumed that at least 50 percent pregnant women are likely to have low blood levels of pyridoxine and presumably would benefit from supplementation. Although an improved diet may be sufficient to raise the blood levels of the vitamin to the norm, the quantities in food are not particularly high and the vitamin itself is likely to be needed. A daily intake of at least 10mg of pyridoxine has been calculated to be needed by a pregnant woman if the metabolism is to be maintained at the same level as that of a non-pregnant female of the same age. This cannot be obtained from the diet which is why the table below does not quote it.

There are other possible benefits of vitamin supplementation to a pregnant woman in addition to ensuring she is not marginally deficient. There is good evidence from various clinical trials that vitamin supplementation during pregnancy is associated with a lower than predicted incidence of the disease spina bifida in women who have already given birth to an afflicted child. No one is quite sure yet if one or more vitamins are involved in increasing the chances of spina bifida when they are deficient, but folic acid is believed to be specifically protective against the condition. Large scale trials recently reported appear to establish that folic acid may have a role in preventing spina bifida. An extra daily intake of 400µg is sufficient. Larger doses have to be prescribed. Meanwhile, it does appear to be a sensible precaution for any pregnant woman to ensure that her daily intake of all vitamins is adequate, either by carefully considering her diet or by taking a low-level all-round multivitamin preparation.

PREGNANCY

VITAMIN	AUS	CAN	NZ	UK	FAO-USA	WHO
VIT A µg	750	900	750	750	1000	750
VIT D µg	10	5.0	10	10	10	2-5
VIT E mg	–	7.0	13.5	–	10	–
VIT C mg	60	50	60	60	80	60
THIAMINE mg	1.2	1.2	1.2	1.0	1.4	1.0
RIBOFLAVIN mg	1.5	1.5	2.5	1.6	1.5	1.5
NICOTINIC ACID mg	19	15	18	18	15	16.8
PYRIDOXINE mg	2.6	2.0	2.5	–	2.6	–
FOLIC ACID µg	400	250	500	300	800	600
VIT B12 µg	3.0	4.0	4.0	–	4.0	5.0

VITAMIN	BREAST–FEEDING					
	AUS	CAN	NZ	UK	FAO-USA	WHO
VIT A µg	1200	1400	1200	750	1200	1200
VIT D µg	10	5.0	10	10	10	10
VIT E mg	–	8.0	13.5	–	11	–
VIT C mg	60	60	60	60	100	60
THIAMINE mg	1.3	1.5	1.3	1.1	1.6	1.1
RIBOFLAVIN mg	1.7	1.7	2.5	1.8	1.7	1.7
NICOTINIC ACID mg	22	25	21	21	18	18.2
PYRIDOXINE mg	3.3	2.6	2.5	–	2.5	–
FOLIC ACID µg	300	250	400	300	500	500
VIT B12 µg	2.5	3.5	4.0	–	4.0	4.5

Do you take the Contraceptive Pill?

More than 100 publications have now appeared in the medical press on the influence of oral contraceptives on the vitamin status of the women taking them. As oral contraceptives are long-term drugs – a woman can take them continually for many years – vitamin deficiencies can develop insidiously until they manifest themselves in various ways. Supplementation taken at sensible levels can help prevent deficiencies and hence reduce the chances of adverse effects.

There is good evidence that the body tissues of women taking the contraceptive pill are unsaturated with respect to vitamin C. This is reflected in higher excretion rates of the vitamin in the urine of these women compared to those levels in women using other forms of contraception. The vitamin C levels in the blood of those on the 'pill' are invariably lower than those women who are not and it is highly significant that it takes 500 mg vitamin C daily for treated women to reach the same blood levels as those who are not treated taking only 50 mg vitamin C daily. This suggests that the ingredients of the 'pill' cause increased turnover of the vitamin or perhaps may reduce the efficiency of its absorption. If you do decide to take 500mg or more of vitamin C while on the 'pill', make sure this vitamin is taken at least four hours after the 'pill' to ensure that the vitamin does not increase the absorption of the oestrogen component of the 'pill' to unacceptable levels.

Many of the B vitamins are also affected by the ingredients of the contraceptive pill and of these vitamins B6 or pyridoxine appear to be the most significant. The reason is that the depression often associated with the use of oral contraceptive appears to be a drug-related phenomenon that manifests itself through a reduction of pyridoxine blood levels. About one in twenty of women taking oral contraceptive become depressed with a characteristic pattern of lethargy, pessimism, anxiety, lack of sexual interest and a tendency to cry easily.

It now appears that this depression is due to interference by the synthetic highly potent oestrogen in the contraceptive pill with the normal chemical reactions in the brain. Normally certain brain substances are produced from the amino acid tryptophane under the influence of vitamin B6. However, 80 percent of women taking an oral contraceptive have an abnormal metabolism of tryptophane resulting in lowered production of the brain substance serotonin. This change in metabolism increases the body's requirement for pyridoxine so that more is needed than is the case in someone not taking the 'pill'.

The suggestion that the depression in the 'pill' takers is due to a deficiency of pyridoxine has been amply confirmed by trials indicating that the vitamin alone can reverse this depression. Women who developed the condition were treated with either pyridoxine or a dummy tablet and their response was assessed. Of 22 women tested, 11 had evidence of vitamin B6 deficiency in their blood and all of them lost the symptoms of depression when treated with the vitamin but not with the dummy tablets. In the 11 women who had no sign of deficiency of the vitamin in the blood; none responded to either pyridoxine or the dummy tablets. The vitamin B extra intakes needed to get over the depression induced by the contraceptive pill varied, but at least 25mg daily can be regarded as the norm.

Other B vitamins reduced by the action of the ingredients of the contraceptive pill include riboflavin, thiamine and vitamin B12. Supplementary intakes needed to restore the normal vitamin status of those women taking it have been calculated as thiamine 5mg; riboflavin 10mg; vitamin B12 4µg. Folic acid levels may be affected as well but fewer women show reduced blood levels of this vitamin. A daily supplement of 300μg should suffice to restore the body to normal. Nicotinic acid requirements from the diet may be reduced because the amino acid tryptophane is diverted to making this instead of being used in synthesis of brain substances in the absence of vitamin B6. However, as the tryptophane made within the body is normalised by vitamin B6 therapy, nicotinic acid synthesis also reaches norrnal levels and the balance between dietary and internal sources of nicotinic acid is restored.

The fat-soluble vitamin A may increase in concentration in the blood in those taking oral contraceptives, perhaps by virtue of an increase in the specific protein that binds the vitamin. This has little significance and can be ignored. What cannot be ignored is the reduced vitamin E levels in the blood that are a feature in those taking the 'pill'. As much as 200 i.u. of vitamin E daily may be required to restore normal values. There is no evidence for a reduction in vitamin D, or K, or the B vitamins pantothenic acid and biotin.

Unless the vitamin deficiencies induced by the contraceptive pill are remedied, the consequences may be serious. Typical signs of deficiency are a general malaise and depression together with increased susceptibility to infections and skin problems. These were the most common signs of deficiency found in a survey of 46,000 women who were taking the 'pill' in Britain. In addition there are several reports of adverse psychiatric, skin and blood side effects of oral contraceptives which responded to specific vitamin therapy. It has also been suggested that the prevalence of thrombosis in these women may be related to vitamin deficiency, with specific reference to vitamin E. All of these results would suggest that any woman taking the contraceptive pill should be aware of possible vitamin deficiencies which are easily overcome by simple supplementation.

Are you convalescing?

Anyone who has suffered an illness or is recovering from an operation is likely to be mildly deficient in vitamins because of a variety of factors. Illness usually gives rise to loss of appetite so the food eaten is reduced and this is parallelled by lowered vitamin intakes in the diet. In addition, the metabolism or excretion of some vitamins may be increased. A prime example is where the blood level of vitamin C drops dramatically at the commencement of an illness, particularly when the complaint is due to an infection.

If the illness is associated with the gastro-intestinal tract, as well as the possibility that normal food intakes are restricted, then the absorption of vitamins may be curtailed. This is highly significant when the condition is associated with fat malabsorption since this, in turn, will adversely affect the uptake of the fat-soluble vitamins. Vitamin A is of paramount importance in strengthening the body's resistance to infection yet many illnesses cause rapid depletion of the vitamin. Blood and tissue levels of the vitamin must, therefore, be maintained and in the absence of dietary supplies supplementation must be sought.

The deficiency of vitamins induced by the nature of the illness and a reduced food intake can be exacerbated by any medical treatment used to treat the complaint. Many drugs, as we have seen previously can have a deleterious effect upon the vitamin status of the body by preventing absorption of the essential micronutrients; by causing excessive excretion of them; by reducing their activity and neutralizing their effects. Most drugs are perhaps only used for short periods of time but they can still reduce vitamin levels sufficient to cause a mild deficiency. This in turn, of course, may slow down the rate of recovery from the illness. The rule in any period of convalescence is therefore to restore the vitamin balance of the body as quickly as possible and supplementation, combined with a good diet, is usually essential.

When the body has been damaged either by accidental injury or a surgical operation, certain vitamins are essential to speed up the healing process. Lack of vitamins C and E, for example, will slow down the rate of healing. Both vitamins should be taken before an impending operation in order to build up body levels and also during the period of con-valescence to maintain these levels. Daily intakes of 400 i.u. vitamin E and 500mg vitamin C should suffice.

The vitamin B complex will also be severely depleted during many illnesses and should be taken at moderate levels. In addition, the mineral zinc which complements the action of many vitamins is essential during the post-operation period. Zinc, amongst other functions, is needed to release vitamin A from its reserves in the liver and hence harness its power to help the body recover from medical and surgical illnesses.

Do you smoke and/or drink?

Those twin habits, smoking tobacco and drinking alcohol, have more in common than the problems encountered when they are taken in excess. They both have a deleterious effect upon the vitamin status of the body. In addition, some of these ill-effects are due to a poisonous substance called acetaldehyde which is not only present in tobacco smoke but is produced from alcohol by the body's own metabolic processes. It is not generally realised that when alcohol is drunk, only about 5 percent of it is excreted as such in the expired air and in the urine. The rest is burned to produce energy via the ordinary metabolic cycles functioning within the body.

As acetaldehyde is the first substance produced from alcohol on this metabolic pathway, and as it is a poisonous substance, its presence in the body is usually of a transitory nature. Similarly, when taken into the blood from tobacco smoke via the lungs, acetaldehyde is normally quickly disposed of. However, the vitamins needed to burn off the acetaldehyde are those which are destroyed to the greater degree by it so when these vitamins are deficient, the ability of the body to dispose of acetaldehyde, from either source, is severely curtailed. Let us now look at those vitamins found to be affected by smoking and drinking.

There have been many reports indicating a possible association between cigarette smoking and ascorbic acid (vitamin C) deficiency. One study compared 154 non-smokers with 100 smokers and showed that plasma vitamin C decreased progressively with increased cigarette consumption. A paper in *Nutrition Today* reported evidence that smokers tended to show lowered utilization of vitamin C with less storage and higher excretion than in non-smokers. The author concluded that smokers would need twice as much vitamin C intake as non-smokers to maintain comparable blood levels. The whole relationship between smoking and vitamin C has been reviewed and the evidence available suggested there may be a good case for the preventative and possibly therapeutic use of ascorbic acid in combating some of the untoward effects of heavy smoking. The drinker of alcohol is also prone to vitamin C deficiency.

Vitamin B6 is another essential food factor that has been found to be at risk in smokers and drinkers. One study compared smoking and non-smoking human males and showed that the presence of nicotine in cigarette smoke reduced the blood levels of vitamin B6. Another study implicated the carbon monoxide of cigarette smoke in the destruction of vitamin B6 in the body leading to low levels in the blood. The blood disorders produced by alcohol have been reported in the *American Journal of Medicine* where B6 deficiency and deficiencies of other vitamins were found in the blood. There was no clear indication whether alcohol produced the deficiency by causing malabsorption of the vitamins or by causing a direct toxic action on the liver. Others have made similar observations.

Lowered blood levels of thiamine produced by drinkers of alcohol have been confirmed by many researchers who performed their studies using radioactive thiamine in their patients. They showed that alcohol interferes with vitamin B1 utilization by the liver and causes decreased absorption of the vitamin from the gastro-intestinal system.

The effect of constituents of tobacco smoke on the enzyme systems of man has also been studied and the evidence indicated that inhibitors in smoke deactivate sulphur-hydrogen groups needed in the defence mechanisms of the body and so reduce its resistance to toxic compounds. The relevance of replacement of SH compounds such as the amino acid to cysteine to restore body protection was therefore clear. Evidence is also accumulating on the effect of the mineral zinc on man's tolerance to ingested alcohol. Zinc is an essential component of the enzyme-detoxicating system for alcohol, but its levels appear to decrease with increasing intake of alcohol.

There is thus ample evidence that the inhalation of tobacco smoke and the ingestion of alcohol may put the individual at risk with reference to certain essential food constituents.

It is well established that one of the most irritating components of tobacco smoke is acetaldehyde. Drinking alcohol also causes the blood level of acetaldehyde to rise. The ill effects of acetaldehyde are seen in the recognised medical treatment of alcoholics where a drug is given deliberately to stop the further detoxification of acetaldehyde produced from alcohol. If alcohol is drunk after the drug has been taken, the ill-effects are so intense as to discourage further drinking. Under ordinary conditions of smoking and drinking the prime consideration is therefore the removal of the acetaldehyde inhaled or produced from alcohol. Nicotine is another major toxic constituent of tobacco smoke that must be removed.

Experimental evidence has indicated that a combination of vitamin C, cysteine and glucose has a better antidotal effect against nicotine and acetaldehyde than vitamin C alone. A combination of vitamin C and cysteine was found to be the best detoxicating mixture against nicotine. A combination of vitamin C, thiamine (vitamin B1) and cysteine was the best detoxicant of acetaldehyde produced by smoking and drinking. When guinea-pigs were given nicotine in tobacco smoke, vitamin C absorption was delayed and reduced. Like man, guinea-pigs rely on extraneous sources of vitamin C since neither can make it.

This means, therefore, that the very food constituents that are required for dealing with the toxic products resulting from smoking and drinking are exactly those that are likely to be deficient in individuals who smoke and/or drink. In addition there is also the possibility of low levels of vitamin B6 and zinc. To ensure that adequate quantities of these constituents are available to the smoker and the drinker they should take a vitamin C supplement (500mg); vitamin B1 (20mg); vitamin B6 (5mg); and zinc (4mg) daily. The best way to avoid a hangover is to take this combination before drinking, while drinking, and most importantly just before sleep. The detoxicating effect of the mineral and vitamins will function while asleep.

Smokers would, in addition, be advised to take beta-carotene daily at a level of 15mg. This substance has been shown in animal experiments to protect the lungs against the cancer-inducing substances in tobacco smoke. At this level, beta-carotene is harmless and can be taken on a regular basis indefinitely. Studies on its protective effect against lung and other cancers are being undertaken at present in human beings but in view of its low toxicity, it is worth a smoker taking beta-carotene regularly even though the question of its action against lung cancer in man has not yet been resolved.

Vitamin A appears to protect the body against certain cancers, including those of the lung, but it may not be as efficient as beta-carotene. In addition, there is much less chance of toxic reactions from beta-carotene than from vitamin A with its high intake required. Beta-carotene is therefore the preferred prophylactic against lung cancer induced by smoking. However, the best preventative remains not to smoke tobacco at all.

Are you slimming?

It has been estimated that some 50 percent of people in the West are over-weight. From the number of slimming regimes available and the advice given by experts (and others) it is obvious that removal of excess weight constantly occupies the thoughts of many people. Here we are talking about overweight due to over-eating. We are not concerned with white fat, brown fat, slow burners, fat burners or any of the other hypothetical concepts put forward to explain why some individuals are overweight. Nor shall we consider excessive weight due to hormonal upsets or other medical problems or medical treatment, all of which are best left to the practitioner. We shall discuss first why people who eat too much are overweight, and then consider the hazards that many encounter when embarking upon a diet eaten with the prime purpose of reducing calorie intake, but with little attention to the requirements of those other essential nutrients, vitamins and minerals.

The body requires only so much energy to function effectively each day, represented by a basic amount necessary for essential life processes, plus a variable amount that depends upon the physical activity of the individual. Even the basic requirements vary amongst people and depend upon age, sex, height, body weight, mental activity and temperament. Basic requirements decrease with age after 25 or so years, and it is the fact that these are less, but food intake remains unaltered and contributes to middle-age spread.

Food intake is energy intake because all food is capable of being converted into energy. When food that is eaten is not being converted into energy, it is stored within the body to be used at some later date. The storage of energy within the body is achieved in the main by the laying down of fat. Some is stored as animal starch or glycogen, particularly in the liver and muscles, but this should be regarded as first-line reserves and is of no consequence in producing a condition of overweight.

Fat storage, of course, has other functions. It serves to act as an insulator against the cold and it is deposited around essential internal organs such as the kidney where it acts as a protective barrier. Fat is also nature's way of saving energy 'for a rainy day'. The conservation of energy as fat is of prime importance to wild animals as they have to eat when they can and have no guarantee of regular meals. They are able to live off their fat reserves until the next feed, which can be hours or, more likely, days away. Most human beings have no such problems. Their three meals a day are virtually guaranteed and too often food intake is geared to appetite rather than to necessity. Small wonder then that energy intake exceeds energy output, with the result that the difference is laid down as body fat. We are laying down reserves of energy with little chance of ever using them. Body weight must increase under these circumstances.

It is important to realise that the three food constituents, carbohydrate, fat and protein, can all be converted by the body into fat. Many diets use the high protein concept where carbohydrate and fat intake are curtailed but lots of protein is eaten. This is fine up to a point but it must be remembered that gram for gram protein supplies 4.00 calories compared to 3.75 calories for carbohydrate. Excess protein is just as liable to be laid down as fat as are starch and sugars. Fat of course, contributes the higher energy at 9 calories per gram, but don't forget alcohol at 7 calories per gram. Hence the ideal diet is balanced in these three basic food constituents but if this intake is reduced, other problems are introduced which are concerned with those essential food constituents, vitamins and minerals.

Foods vary tremendously in their content of vitamins and minerals; this is why only a balanced, good quality and varied diet will supply all the essential nutrients for health. Most vitamins are sensitive chemical compounds which means that any excess cooking or bad storage of foods can often destroy them irreversibly. Minerals cannot be destroyed but they can be removed from foods by over-refining and processing; they are often discarded in water used for cooking, and they are liable to be irreversibly bound to other food constituents, making them unavailable to the body. Minerals in our food must ultimately come from the soil, yet it is known that this varies widely in its mineral content and is often lacking in essential trace elements. It is hoped that a normal intake of food taken from a wide variety of sources and cooked expertly will supply all the necessary vitamins and minerals. How then can someone on a slimming diet with a restricted food intake hope to obtain their full requirements of these nutrients? The answer is that they are unlikely to. In fact, slimmers are now recognized officially as a group of the population who may be liable to vitamin and mineral deficiency when their slimming regimes are undertaken without professional advice.

Just how deficient in vitamins and minerals could an individual on a slimming diet be? If we take an average calorie requirement from a normal diet for an adult female to be say, 2,300 calories and an adult male to need 2,900 calories, we can assume that the amount of food to supply this would also supply the daily requirements of vitamins and minerals. When these people reduce their intake of food energy to the conventional 1,000 calories there must also be a concomitant decrease in their intake of the essential nutrients. Unfortunately, however, the body requirements for vitamins and minerals are the same regardless of the calorie intake. The only exception to this is thiamine or vitamin B1 whose requirements are related to carbohydrate intake; the more carbohydrate eaten the more vitamin B1 is needed. All other vitamins are necessary for health in minimum quantities that have no relationship to energy intake.

Individual items of food have varying contents of the various vitamins and minerals and there is a risk that in avoiding some high calorie foods when on a slimming diet there is a greater risk of deficiency, in particular vitamins and minerals. Potatoes, for example, are our main source of vitamin C, not because they are the richest source of the vitamin but due essentially to the large bulk eaten. Unfortunately, potatoes are also usually the first item of food that a slimmer will remove from the diet since they are an excellent source of calories. The slimmer should therefore look to low calorie alternatives rich in vitamin C such as unsweetened natural fruit juice and raw fruit and lightly-cooked green vegetables.

Cereals are rich in the vitamin B complex yet slimmers tend to avoid these foods because of their high carbohydrate content. Bread is an important source of the vitamin B group and is another example of a food usually taken in large quantity that contributes a large proportion of these vitamins to the body.

Where then are the slimmers, who usually cut down on bread, going to obtain their B vitamins? Most meats and particularly liver are very rich in the B vitamins, so this presents no problem to the meat eater. However, the vegetarian can look to a variety of foods. Fortunately, whole raw nuts are a rich source of all these vitamins (apart from vitamin B12) and remember that each ounce will contribute a good share of the daily protein requirements. Eggs, of course, are a complete food that should feature in any slimmer's diet. Dried fruit will also yield useful amounts of the B group without making too large a hole in the calorie count. Green vegetables are also useful sources but it is important not to destroy the vitamins by overcooking.

It is unlikely that these vegetable foods will give you sufficient vitamin B12 and it is essential to ensure some intake of meats or dairy products on a slimming diet to ensure adequate amounts of this vitamin. The liver carries useful stores of vitamin B12 in most individuals but on any long-term slimming regime these could be depleted if the intake of meat and dairy products is curtailed. Most dairy products are avoided by slimmers because of their high fat content so it is important to make sure of one's vitamin B12 requirements by taking some meat.

Vegetarians may wish to obtain their B12 from cheeses at the expense of their calorie intake but a supplement is the safest and easiest way to ensure their B12 requirements.

Folic acid is unlikely to present a problem to the slimmer as the richest sources are green leaf vegetables and salads – both are foods that tend to be eaten in large quantities on a calorie-restricted diet. Liver, which should also feature in a slimmer's diet, is high in folic acid and has the advantage of being rich in the type of folic acid that can be used by man.

The vitamins most at risk in slimmers are the fat soluble A, D and E. This is because by their very nature they are associated with fats and oils that the slimmer tends to avoid. During winter months the food is the more important source of vitamin D and is found in dairy products, fish and liver. A low intake of these will reflect in low body levels of the vitamin. In the absence of dairy products a daily supplement is advisable. There should however be no problem in the summer as long as sufficient sunlight is allowed to fall on the skin, since the action of ultra-violet rays actually produces vitamin D in the skin. Switching from full cream milk to the skimmed variety will also deprive the slimmer of the fat soluble vitamins which must then be obtained from other sources.

The meat eater should derive ample vitamin A from liver as long as this is taken as part of the diet. Fish is also an excellent source of both vitamins A and D. The vegetarian will, it is hoped, obtain his or her vitamin A from carotenes that are found in plants, but remember that not all carotenes are precursors of the vitamin. Carrots, spinach, broccoli and Brussels sprout are particularly rich in carotene that will give rise to vitamin A.

Vitamin E occurs in the highest concentration in vegetable oils and, although the slimmer may be wary of these in view of their high calorie content, some should feature in every diet. In addition, these oils supply the essential polyunsaturated fatty acids that are needed in many body functions. A daily intake of oils will therefore ensure adequate vitamin E and vitamin F (another name for polyunsaturated fatty acids). Vitamin E is widely distributed in many foods but its concentration is low and when the actual quantity of food consumed is reduced as in the slimmer, a low intake of vitamin E follows. The simplest way to take vitamin E is in capsules that contribute not only the vitamin but also the polyunsaturated fatty acids. The calorific value of these capsules is so low as to be negligible.

Meat and fish are generally regarded as suitable for slimmers and fortunately these foods are good sources of many of the vitamins mentioned. However, for a variety of reasons such foods are not always eaten by the slimmer in sufficient quantity to yield the full complement of vitamins necessary. In addition, meat and fish are usually low in vitamins C and E, both of which are required in the highest quantities amongst the vitamins. Therefore, a balanced diet should be sought to incorporate other foods rich in these vitamins. Even so, on a daily intake of 1,000 calories there is the possibility of mild deficiency. Vegetarian slimmers are most likely to obtain a balanced vitamin intake but this is tempered by a lower bulk of food than is usual and their total intake is likely to be less.

The simplest insurance for anyone undergoing a slimming regime is a daily supplement of all the vitamins necessary to sustain life. Choose any one of the many multivitamin preparations available, any one of which per day will give sufficient vitamins without reference to those taken in the diet. We know that vitamins are essential in the processes of burning food to give energy, in the interconversion of foods and to burn off that unsightly fat that is the aim of every slimmer. A deficiency of vitamins must reflect in a less efficient system for disposing of excess weight. Minerals are just as important to health as vitamins and they act together with vitamins in controlling the metabolism of the body. We rely upon food as a source of minerals so that these too may be prone to deficiency as the amount of food eaten is reduced during slimming bouts. The minerals required in relatively large amounts such as calcium and phosphorus are present in high concentration in dairy products but these foods are often ignored by the slimmer. Shellfish contribute reasonable amounts of calcium and phosphorus but they would not be acceptable to the vegetarian. Bread and cereals are good sources of calcium but these too are foods generally avoided by slimmers. Vegetables must therefore be the most important source of calcium and phosphorus to the slimmer. Our skeleton acts as a rich reservoir of calcium but during prolonged periods of slimming the withdrawal of calcium and phosphorus from bone could tend to weaken it. In the absence of dairy products, then, a supplement of calcium must be sought.

Magnesium is widely distributed in all foods but the reduction of calories to 1,000 or so per day must adversely affect the intake of this mineral. Low magnesium in the body leads to irritability, depression, mild mental problems and muscular weakness. How often are these conditions associated with the slimmer! Magnesium is best taken as a supplement in the form of dolomite tablets. These supply calcium as well and the two minerals are in the same ratio in dolomite as in the required intake from food. They are calorie-free and dissolve in stomach acid to ensure good absorption.

Even on normal diets supplying the average calorie requirement, iron is often at risk in view of its poor absorption. The possibility of deficiency must therefore increase on a reduced calorie intake. Again the meat eater has some advantage over his or her vegetarian counterpart because the iron from meat is better absorbed than that from vegetables. Under normal circumstances this does not matter because the vegetarian makes up in quantity of vegetable foods what they lack in quality, but a reduction in food intake will almost certainly give rise to iron deficiency. In the female of child-bearing age this deficiency may be exacerbated by menstrual loss of iron and the chances of full replacement on a slimming diet are remote. Therefore, the slimmer must choose foods with a high iron content – usually of animal origin – but failing this they should seek a supplement. Iron from iron salts is notoriously difficult to absorb so that the quantity of salts taken are far in excess of that needed. Iron amino acid chelates are the nearest equivalent to the iron presented in meat (although of vegetable origin) with the result that absorption is superior to that of iron salts.

Zinc is another mineral assuming more and more importance as research continues and it tends to be associated with high protein foods. Hence, any slimming diet that is low in protein-rich constituents will be deficient in zinc.

There is considerable doubt as to whether conventional diets provide sufficient zinc so the chances of deficiency from a calorie-reduced diet are enhanced. Sea foods are particularly rich in zinc and they contribute other minerals from the sea as well as protein at the expense of a few calories. Nuts are also good sources of zinc so that the non-fish eater can obtain some of their requirements from these.

The simplest way to ensure a good intake of trace minerals daily, particularly whilst slimming, is to take kelp. Kelp is dried seaweed that has concentrated in it all of the minerals of the sea, probably the richest source of minerals of any area in the world. In addition, kelp is an excellent source of iodine which has a very important role in the body. Iodine is a constituent of thyroxine, the hormone from the thyroid gland that controls body metabolism. Low iodine levels mean a sluggish metabolism which is the last condition a slimmer would want. By ensuring an adequate iodine intake, a slimmer can make certain that the body has every chance to metabolise its food and, more importantly, turn excess fat into energy. In addition, the other minerals in kelp are essential ingredients in the enzymes necessary for the metabolic conversion of food and fat into energy.

There is little doubt that people will continue to undertake slimming diets without medical supervision for a long time to come. As long as they are aware of the need for the following they should come to no harm:

1. A minimum intake of calories, usually 800-1000 daily

2. A minimum intake of protein, usually 40-60 grams daily

3. A supplemental intake of all vitamins and minerals.

At least it is possible to ensure an adequate supply of vitamins and minerals using supplements that yield only a negligible quantity of calories. Supplementation removes some of the problems associated with dieting. All that is left then is an awareness of protein intake and the pleasure of calorie-counting.

Do you fall into one of these other categories?

Those under stress

Some years ago animal experiments indicated that during periods of stress the requirements for the vitamin B complex and vitamin C increased. In any animal, under stress conditions, the body reacts by producing hormones from the glands that enable it to overcome the effects of that stress. Vitamins B and C and certain minerals are essential in the production of these hormones and so they contribute to the animal's defence against stress. A similar situation was observed in the American astronauts. During the early space flights it was discovered that although the men appeared to have adequate intakes of all the vitamins in their food, they were not sufficient for the great physical and mental stress that the astronauts underwent. On return to Earth, their blood levels of vitamins were dangerously low.

Particularly susceptible were vitamin B and C, but also vitamin E. In fact, vitamin E levels were so low that all of the astronauts developed anaemia whilst on the flight, due mainly to massive haemolysis (breakdown) of red blood cells. In later flights all the vitamin intakes were increased and the biochemical problems did not arise. Not many of us will undergo space flights but what was learned from these pioneers may help us in overcoming the stress of life.

Menstruating women

We have seen that women who take the contraceptive pill are inducing in themselves an increased requirement for vitamin B6. This is due to a direct action of the synthetic female sex hormones in the preparation, but mainly the oestrogenic component, that cause increased usage of vitamin B6 and probably also reduce its absorption from the food.

A similar phenomenon is seen in some women who are not taking the contraceptive pill but still suffer the same sort of symptoms, known as Premenstrual Syndrome (PMS), ten days or so before their period is due to start. It is likely that over-production of oestrogens or reduced synthesis of the other sex hormone progesterone by the female is the prime cause of PMS. Treatment is therefore aimed at overcoming any vitamin deficiency that contributes to the hormone imbalance.

Vitamin B6 helps some women who suffer from premenstrual tension. In a trial carried out at St. Thomas's Hospital in London, vitamin B6 supplementation was compared to hormone treatment over a period of seven months. Significant improvement was seen in those treated with hormones in terms of premenstrual irritability, depression and swelling of the abdomen. An overall improvement in 73 percent of these patients was noted with this treatment. A comparable group of women was given vitamin B6 in 100mg dose daily. At this level there was an overall improvement of symptoms in 63 percent of the women. The results suggest that perhaps vitamin B6 should be the primary treatment of premenstrual tension as it is successful, natural, and lacks side-effects at this dose.

Simple supplementation with vitamin B6 will help many women suffering from PMS but there are always some who will not respond or whose symptoms are only partially relieved by the vitamin. In these cases another natural approach is often recommended which is not strictly replacing a vitamin deficiency but nevertheless has a vitamin-like action.

At one time the polyunsaturated fatty acids (also known as essential fatty acids) were known as vitamin F but as their mode of action became clearer it was realised that the most important member was *linoleic acid*. The designation vitamin F for this acid was eventually discarded as, although it was essential and could be obtained only from the food, its daily requirements were too high to define it as a true vitamin. Nevertheless, the term vitamin F still persists in some parts of the world.

Linoleic acid has many functions within the body, but the one that concerns us here is that of being the starting material in the production of prostaglandins. These are important hormones that control many of the essential life processes and they are produced only in the body from dietary linoleic acid. To be made into prostaglandins, linoleic acid must first be converted to gamma linoleic acid and this step appears to be the main stumbling block in conditions where prostaglandin synthesis is curtailed. For example, women who suffer PMS appear, first, to have a polyunsaturated fatty acid deficiency and, second, to be unable to produce enough gamma linoleic acid to satisfy their needs. Treatment of

PMS is therefore aimed at supplying both polyunsaturated fatty acids (particularly linoleic) and gamma linoleic acid.

Oil of evening primrose is obtained from the seeds of that plant and it is one of the richer sources of both polyunsaturated fatty acids and of gamma linoleic acid. Hence, by taking the oil (usually in capsule form) for the ten days or so before a period is due, a female can ensure she has adequate intakes of linoleic and gamma linoleic acids. If her PMS is due to lack of these, supplementation with the acids will relieve her symptoms. This has been amply proved in many clinical trials.

Hence any female who suffers PMS can take vitamin B6 and/or oil of evening primrose as a perfectly natural treatment for her symptoms. This represents a self-help natural alternative to the hormone treatment prescribed by her medical practitioner and is one devoid of possible side-effects.

Asian immigrants

Members of some immigrant populations often avoid certain foods for religious reasons and so create an imbalance in their nutritional intake.

Concerns have been expressed in recent years over the re-appearance of rickets due to vitamin D deficiency among Asian immigrants in the UK. The disorder is due to inadequate intake of vitamin D, plus failure in the formation of the vitamins from 7-dehydrocholesterol in the skin thanks to a lack of sunlight and the presence of pigmentation.

The obvious remedy is supplementary vitamin D in the diet, and a Government study group has decided that this is the best way to overcome deficiency. However, many Asians are vegetarians, so that good sources like cod liver oil and liver are not acceptable. They can however seek other sources such as those from irradiated yeast. Nonetheless, simply giving extra vitamin D may not be the complete answer. The recent study of white children in the UK, quoted earlier provided evidence that those who had a seaside holiday during the previous summer had a higher blood level of vitamin D during the winter than those who had not. In both children and adults, vitamin supplementation increased blood levels, but not up to the level of those exposed to sunshine all those months previously.

The answer may, therefore, be a change in diet that supplies vitamin D;

supplementation in the winter months, and a more prolonged exposure to sunshine when this is available.

Those who live alone

Another group of the population at risk from vitamin and mineral deficiencies is that consisting of those living alone. These people are often elderly and hence suffer from the same dietary problems as those mentioned previously. In addition, however, loss of a partner often induces a reluctance to cook food for one so that cheap, refined carbohydrates and simple beverages are relied upon as a staple diet. Often these people will rely upon institutional or supplied meals (in which excessive vitamin and mineral loss may be prevalent) for their dietary needs. An official study which was undertaken in 1972 found that men living alone had lower intakes of food and hence essential nutrients than those living with a wife or family.

Even younger people are not immune as they will often rely upon quick and easy-to-cook convenience foods that are not always guaranteed full nutritional value. Students fall into this category as pointed out in an official comprehensive study carried out in 1974. Intakes of vitamin C, B1 and B2 varied tremendously amongst students and the contributing factors were believed to be reliance on institutional meals, poor self catering and financial inability to purchase a good all-round nutritious diet.

Supplementation with a good all-round multivitamin preparation, whilst not replacing an improved diet, will at least ensure the minimum daily requirement of vitamins without reference to those in the food.

Children

Children are notorious as faddy eaters and nothing is more calculated to put a child off healthy nutrition than telling them that food 'is good for them'. Children often do not eat the right foods because they do not like them and instead prefer to fill up on sweet or savoury snacks that add calories but little else. Unfortunately, lack of vitamins and/or minerals during the growing period can adversely affect growth and development, both mental and physical. Medical studies on children in poor communities in the Middle East indicated that a lack of zinc was a direct cause of reduced sexual, physical and mental development. Adding extra zinc to the diet normalised their complete development. Similarly, lack of vitamin E in the diet of children can retard growth and induce anaemia, conditions that were only cured by supplementing the diet with vitamin E.

Athletes

Athletes in general have a greater energy requirement due to their physical exertions, but it is important for them to ensure an adequate vitamin and mineral intake to parallel those extra dietary calories. Too often the additional food an athlete takes during training or competition consists of glucose sweets and drinks and pure protein which are calories devoid of minerals and vitamins. Many sportsmen obtain at least part of their dietary intake from institutional sources like colleges, works or office restaurants, with the danger that such overcooked foods may be deficient in vitamins, particularly vitamin C. This vitamin is important in the production of body hormones which are required in higher concentration during excessive physical activity. The vitamin B complex which is concerned in the conversion of food into energy may wisely be taken during intense physical activity. Both vitamins B1 and B2 appear to be essential in recovery from fatigue. Excessive perspiration during athletic pursuits leads to loss of minerals in the sweat that can only be replaced in the food.

Blood supply to muscles must be efficient to ensure they receive a constant supply of oxygen, glucose and other nutrients. In addition, of course, the blood from the muscles must also be adequate to take away the waste products of muscle metabolism, many of which can be toxic if allowed to build up. For this reason, many athletes take extra vitamin E, up to 1,000 i.u. daily, to ensure that the supply in the blood is sufficient. The vitamin not only increases the efficiency of oxygen carriage in the blood and its uptake by the muscles but dilates the blood vessels to ensure adequate blood reaches the muscles.

How to cope?

The important question now arises: How can we overcome these deficiencies?

It would be irresponsible to say, 'Take vitamins, and don't bother about what you eat, drink or smoke'. Eating meals of natural foods that haven't been processed, refined or over-cooked must remain the basis of your vitamin supply. Reducing the amount of alcohol you drink is beneficial to general health. Stopping smoking is probably the most valuable single step towards improved health you can make.

Having said that, there remain all those situations where good eating habits are sabotaged by circumstances, whether of choice – such as slimming – or not, such as being tied to the food served in a hospital, school, company canteen or other institutional catering.

In such circumstances, it is very difficult for the individual to work out where his vitamin intake may be lacking. So the best insurance against nutritional deficiencies is a daily multivitamin preparation, and it must be one rich enough in the vitamins to guarantee an adequate intake for anyone, regardless of their dietary sources. If you drink or smoke or are on 'the pill', no multivitamin preparation is sufficiently potent in individual vitamins to overcome their effects. Specific supplements for these conditions must be sought, although it must be realised that these can only help offset such effects as may be related to vitamin deficiencies caused by these drugs. There is no supplement that can protect you from their other, far-reaching effects on the body.

Finally, if you are on any long-term drug treatment, your doctor should be aware of potential vitamin deficiencies. However, these are very specialised and usually pose no problem with short term medicines. Perhaps we can change a popular quote by saying 'a multivitamin a day', rather than 'an apple a day', is more likely to keep the doctor away.

8 Treating yourself with vitamins

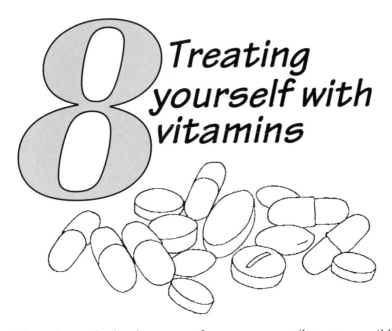

There is no doubt that many factors can contribute to a mild and sometimes temporary deficiency of vitamins, sufficient in some people to cause ill-health and to prevent their living at one hundred percent of their potential. Simple supplementation, often with a general all-round multivitamin preparation or, in the case of specific deficiencies, with the particular vitamin affected is usually enough to overcome problems associated with reduced intakes. When these are a result of poor diet, fairly low potencies of all the vitamins are usually sufficient to insure against any deficiency. However, when the factors inducing deficiency are associated with life styles, medicinal drugs and habits like smoking and drinking, rather higher potencies of the missing vitamins may be needed up to five or even ten times the recommended minimum daily allowances. To these two groups must now be added a third, that of high potency intakes where the vitamin or vitamins are being used for their therapeutic effect in certain clinical conditions.

When the vitamin intake has reached such a low degree that a gross deficiency disease (such as, for example, beriberi, pellagra or scurvy, due respectively to lack of thiamine, nicotinic acid or vitamin C) manifests itself, then diagnosis and treatment become the province of the medical practitioner. Such diseases are rare in this country and in the Western world in general but occasionally they do appear. The symptoms of beriberi, for example, are not uncommon in alcoholics, but when deficiency has reached this stage, it is not suitable for self-treatment and professional help must be sought. This is not to say that anyone who drinks alcohol regularly should not be aware that their vitamin B complex (particularly thiamine) status is at risk, but if they are, regular supplementation with these vitamins, plus vitamin C, should at least ensure that they are unlikely to reach the stage of alcoholic beriberi. In fact, it has been seriously suggested that vitamin B1 should be added to alcoholic drinks to help those who will not help themselves. There is also some evidence that high intakes of the vitamin B complex and vitamin C can help remove the craving for alcohol in chronic alcoholics.

What we are more concerned with in this book is how people who wish to treat themselves with vitamins at high dose can do so safely and successfully. Vitamins will often complement medicinal drug treatments but therapy with these micro nutrients should never be used as a replacement for prescribed drugs without the full knowledge of the doctor prescribing those drugs. Vitamins will not interfere with medicines, with one or two exceptions already noted previously, and indeed both will often function effectively together. You may rest assured, therefore, that the dosage regimes suggested are safe and in the trials where they have been tested, are beneficial. Trials can vary in the way they are carried out but it is accepted that the most meaningful trial is known as double-blind. A double-blind trial compares the effect of the vitamin with a harmless compound (placebo) in a similar presentation in the treatment of the condition. Double-blind simply means that neither the patient nor doctor knows which is which until the end of the trial. In this way the result cannot be influenced by personal bias.

Cancer

VITAMIN A

There are few instances of vitamin A or beta-carotene therapy actually curing an established cancer (a prescribable derivative called retinoic acid has helped in skin cancer) but there are many studies indicating a correlation between body levels of the vitamins and the chances of developing cancer. When blood levels of vitamin A and/or beta-carotene are persistently low, the incidence of cancer increases. This was first illustrated in animal experiments when it was noted that apparently healthy animals which had low body levels of vitamin A were more susceptible to the formation of tumours than those with adequate levels of the vitamin.

Observations on humans have also suggested that low vitamin A or beta-carotene intakes may increase their susceptibility to cancer. Typical is a five-year follow-up study of 8,278 men in Norway. Here, the incidence of confirmed lung cancer and glandular cancers was 4.6 times higher in men classified as having low vitamin A intake. This difference was statistically highly significant and independent of smoking habits. Other studies of blood vitamin A levels, measured as retinol, have demonstrated lower levels in patients with cancer than in control persons without cancer.

A survey, starting in 1975, was carried out as a joint study between Radcliffe Infirmary, Oxford and BUPA Medical Research and reported in *The Lancet* (1980). In a prospective study of about 16,000 men who attended the BUPA Medical Centre for health screening, blood samples were collected and stored at deep freeze temperatures. By the end of 1979, 86 men were identified who had developed cancer. Another 172 men who were alive and without cancer were selected from the remainder of the study population as a control group for comparison. The men in this group were chosen because of similar age and similar smoking habits and because their blood was taken at almost identical times. Vitamin A levels were measured as well as other criteria, such as blood cholesterol. What emerged from the study was that low vitamin A levels were associated with an increased risk of cancer. This association was independent of age, smoking habits and serum cholesterol levels and was greatest for men who developed lung cancer. Their vitamin A levels were only 18 i.u. per 100ml of blood compared with 229 i.uc. per 100ml for the men in control group. The risk of cancer at any body site for men with retinol levels at the lower end of the scale was 2.2. times greater than for those with the higher levels. The conclusion reached was that measures taken to increase serum vitamin A levels in men may lead to a reduction in cancer risk.

A comparable study was carried out on 3,100 patients in Evans County, Georgia in the USA. Low blood levels of vitamin A proved to be associated with an increased incidence of cancer that was independent of age and smoking habits. It was further found that those people who died of lung cancer invariably had lower blood levels not only of vitamin A, but of beta-carotene also, compared to those dying of non-cancer diseases. In these cases, it was also possible to measure the vitamin and its precursor in the liver, and again it was found that reserves of both nutrients were much lower in the cancer victims.

When we look at the relationship between a specific type of tumour, namely lung cancer, and vitamin A intake and smoking habits, a more significant connection emerges. Dr. E. Bjelke reported, in the *International Journal of Cancer*, that when men were matched for equivalent tobacco smoking habits, those with a lower dietary intake of vitamin A had a higher incidence of lung cancer. The main dietary differences between the two groups was a higher consumption of carrots, milk and eggs in those people less prone to lung cancer. All these foods, of course, are excellent sources of vitamin A and carotene. However, other findings emerged from the results. Dietary vitamin A was found to be inversely related to a five year risk of lung cancer among men who were current or former cigarette smokers. After allowing for the number of cigarettes smoked per day, men with lower levels of blood vitamin A, who also ate less quantities of vitamin A and beta carotene-rich foods, had more than 2.5 times the chance of developing lung cancer than those with good intakes of these micro nutrients.

Confirmation that beta-carotene appears to confer a better protective effect against lung cancer than vitamin A was suggested by a study carried out on employees of the Western Electric Company in Chicago, USA. A total of 2,107 men were examined in October 1957 and December 1958 as to their dietary habits, including the taking of vitamin supplements. All the men participating in the trial were re-examined in this manner annually until 1969. Nine years after this the incidence of cancer over the 19 years following the start of the trial was assessed. The results were as follows. Men in the group that comprised the lowest 25 percent of carotene intake had seven times the relative risk of lung cancer as men in the group that made up the highest 25 percent of carotene intake. Among men who had smoked cigarettes for 30 years or more, the relative risk of developing lung cancer was eight times as great for men with low carotene consumption as for those with a high intake of the pro-vitamin.

After analysis of other nutrients in the diet, the authors of the study concluded that the key dietary variable related to risk of lung cancer is carotene. Pre-formed vitamin A and other nutrients provided by their diets were not significantly related to the risk of lung cancer.

The authors conclude that a diet relatively high in beta-carotene may reduce the risk of lung cancer, even among persons who have smoked cigarettes for many years. They emphasise, however, that cigarette smoking increases the risk of other serious diseases such as strokes and coronary thrombosis and there is no evidence that dietary carotene affects the chances of developing these.

Similarly, studies from Israel reported in the *International Journal of Cancer* indicate that there is no protective effect of vitamin A consumption against cancers of the gastro-intestinal tract, but there is a decreased risk of cancer in those who eat beta-carotene rich foods.

We can conclude, therefore, that beta-carotene is preferred to vitamin A as a natural dietary agent to protect against cancer. Even in those with cancer, it is advisable to take extra beta-carotene (13.5mg daily) which may slow down the growth of the cancer. As beta-carotene is much less toxic than vitamin A, the amount suggested will do no harm. It is perhaps significant that fruit and vegetables, both rich in beta-carotene, appear to protect the individual against cancers of the stomach and of the colon.

VITAMIN C

Many studies have found that the lower the amount of vitamin C eaten, the greater the chance of developing cancer. One study in Canada indicated that those with higher regular vitamin C intake in their diets had only 40 percent of the incidences of those with persistently low intake of the vitamin in the same age groups. By increasing the daily intake of dietary vitamin C from 25mg to 125mg there was a 60 percent decrease in the chances of developing cancer. This represents an increase of life expectancy of eleven years. At the same time, it has been observed that cancer sufferers usually have low body levels of vitamin C and their requirements are higher than those not suffering from the disease. The moral would therefore appear to be – ensure an optimal intake of vitamin C daily (say 500-1,000mg) and you could cut down your chance of developing cancer.

Actual therapy with vitamin C in treating cancers has been tried with varying results. Two typical studies are as follows: Ascorbic acid has been shown to be effective against some artificially produced cancers in mice, rats and guinea-pigs but there are very few clinical trials in man. The most comprehensive was that reported by Dr. Ewan Cameron from the Vale of Leven Hospital in Scotland. He treated 100 advanced cancer patients with 10g of ascorbic acid per day (given as sodium ascorbate), and reported that they felt better, had more energy, had better appetites and, in some cases, suffered much less pain. In a few cases their tumours shrank, and in a very small proportion the growth disappeared. The most promising result was an increased average survival time of 293 days. a similar group of advanced cancer patients, who had not received vitamin C treatment had an average survival time of only 38 days. The results, though not outstanding, were promising. A similar study was therefore undertaken by the Mayo Clinic in Rochester, Minnesota, USA. These researchers reported in the *New England Journal of Medicine* that they had treated 60 advanced cancer patients with 10g of vitamin C per day, given as 20 tablets of 500mg each. A comparative group of 63 patients of the same type and stage of cancer, age and sex were given milk sugar tablets to act as a placebo, i.e. an innocuous substance that can have no therapeutic action. There was no difference in survival time of the two groups. About 80 percent of the patients in each group were dead three months after the study began. All but one of the 123 patients were dead within eight months and the one left alive was taking placebo tablets. Even the improvements in symptoms were similar, 63 percent of this category taking vitamin C and 58 percent on milk sugar tablets.

The main difference between the two trials was that the patients in Scotland had not received the strong immunosuppressive drugs that those in USA had been treated with. Dr. Linus Pauling believes this may explain the different responses. He believes that the natural response of the body to vitamin C is weakened by the powerful drugs used in the North American study, most of which reduce the body's natural immunity. The fact remains, however, that in any type of cancer, but particularly those where the local concentration of vitamin C can be high, e.g. gastro intestinal and urinary system cancers, high doses of vitamin C are worth trying. The rule is to take one gram of the vitamin on the first day, two grams on the second and so on up to a maximum of ten grams daily. If the vitamin causes diarrhoea at any level, that potency less one gram should be the dose that is maintained daily. Using this technique it is possible to arrive at one's tolerable level of vitamin C for taking on a regular basis.

Although there is growing epidemiological evidence that antioxidant vitamins and minerals appear to increase resistance of the body to developing certain types of cancers when taken over long periods, there is much less evidence that these nutrients can slow down or even reverse the cancer process. Some examples are given in this chapter but many of the intervention trials i.e. giving specific supplements to people with existing cancer, are still underway and the few results already published do not give firm evidence yet that supplementation alone may help. What is apparent however is that the side effects of cancer therapy whether with drugs (chemotherapy) or with radiation (radiotherapy) can be reduced or avoided by proper supplementation with vitamins and minerals. In addition, there are published studies showing that specific supplementation can complement the action of chemotherapy. This perhaps is not surprising when one considers the way in which anti-cancer drugs function. They are all cytotoxic agents which means that they are designed to stop cell division in cancer cells so that they eventually die. Radiotherapy does the same job but kills the cells with radiation. Unfortunately neither approach is absolutely specific for cancer cells so that normal healthy cells are also adversely affected. The healthy cells so affected most are those of the immunosuppressive system and when this happens the resistance to infections and other ailments is reduced. This resistance in turn depends upon adequate intakes of vitamins and minerals in particular those classed as antioxidants. It is therefore a sensible idea to supplement with these nutrients whilst on chemotherapy and radiotherapy and for some time after these therapies finish. One of the most effective antioxidants is coenzyme Q10 which is not a true vitamin within the definition but it does have vitamin-like properties. A typical intake would be 30mg coenzyme Q10 three times daily. Other antioxidants that may be safely taken are vitamin C (500mg daily); vitamin E (400mg daily); vitamin B complex (10-25mg of each number, apart from folic acid and B12, in combination); folic acid 400µg daily; vitamin B12 100µg daily; beta-carotene 15mg daily and the trace mineral selenium 100-200µg daily. Whilst benefitting the body as a whole, these nutrients will not interfere with the actions of the anti-cancer drugs.

LAETRILE

This substance, incorrectly called vitamin B17, is extracted from apricot kernels and it has been claimed to be of benefit in treating various cancers. It contains organic cyanide which is believed by its proponents to act against the tumour, causing its regression. Unfortunately, it is possible to take too much laetrile which can give rise to cyanide poisoning. For this reason the substance has now been put on the prescription-only list in the UK so it is not suitable for self-treatment.

Skin Diseases

VITAMIN A

The skin-protecting properties of vitamin A are well established but when it was tried in high doses in acne, rosacea and psoriasis, its success rate was variable. At the same time, there were worries about possible side-effects from the megadoses used. In one trial, 18 patients were given up to 200,000 i.e. per day for between 15 and 20 injections. This course was repeated three or five times and the results were promising. Symptoms disappeared in seven patients, improved substantially in nine and improved slightly in two, but side-effects appeared and their extent was such as to cause cessation of the trial after a few months. However, trials such as these did give benefit to some sufferers from skin disease, so research was switched away from vitamin A itself to derivatives with similar or greater positive action but less side-effects. These include retinoic acid but this is not available on general sale.

There are many anecdotal reports of the benefits of relatively low-dose supplementation of vitamin A, (i.e. up to 10,000 i.u. daily) on acne, eczema and psoriasis and other skin complaints. The action of vitamin A is enhanced by simultaneous supplementation with the mineral zinc (up to 15mg daily) probably because one function of this mineral is to ensure adequate uptake of the vitamin by tissues and its release from the liver.

Since acne often appears during puberty, it has been suggested that the sex hormones are involved in its development. We know that vitamin A is necessary for the natural production of sex hormones so it may be acting through these. Whatever the mechanism however, this low dose regime of vitamin A plus zinc has been successful in relieving minor skin complaints in some people.

OIL OF EVENING PRIMROSE

The oil of the Evening Primrose is another natural product claimed to help in clearing up mild skin complaints when taken at the rate of 750 mg daily. The mode of action of this oil is to supply precursors of other important body hormones known as prostaglandins. These, too, may have a role to play in normalizing skin cell formation and again their action may be activated through vitamin A and zinc. The sensible way to approach self-treatment of these skin complaints is to ensure there is no deficiency of any of these factors. Supplementation at the levels recommended will do this, and it is comforting to know that there is no harm at these potencies. In addition, if you can obtain some oil of Evening Primrose cream or ointment, this can be applied directly to the skin lesions and so increase the effect of the oral treatment.

BIOTIN

This member of the vitamin B complex can be used in some cases of scaly dermatitis. It is of particular benefit in babies who develop seborrhoeic dermatitis – a dry scaling of the scalp and face. This is sometimes associated with breast-feeding as human milk is low in biotin. Up to 10mg daily will cure this condition but similar doses are worth trying in other cases of scaly dermatitis. Other skin complaints, alopecia and scalp conditions may also respond to these intakes of biotin which are perfectly safe to take.

Ulcers

VITAMIN B2

Recurrent mouth ulcers have been claimed to be prevented by daily intakes of 20mg or more of vitamin B2. Similar studies on stomach and duodenal ulcers resulted in a less dramatic response, but this was probably because these lesions are a result of many factors, amongst which may be riboflavin deficiency.

Ulceration of the cornea of the eye will sometimes respond to high potency supplementation with vitamin B2. In a study of 47 patients suffering from eye and eyesight problems, six of whom were affected by cataracts, Dr. U. P. Sydenstricker reported in *Prevention* that all disorders were gradually cured with vitamin B2 supplementation. It was essential to carry on with the high riboflavin intake since, when this ceased, the eye complaints returned.

These results parallel those in animals suffering from this condition, but it must be stressed that other B vitamins, like pantothenic acid, may also be involved in prevention of cataracts. Recent research has equated low levels of vitamin C intake throughout life with increased chances of developing cataracts in later life.

VITAMIN A

Vitamin A has a protective effect on mucosal tissue, so it may have the potential for exerting a similar action against gastric ulcer. This hypothesis has been tested in a multi-centre, randomised, controlled trial of vitamin A in 60 patients with chronic gastric ulcers. The trial took place in Hungary and was reported in *The Lancet* towards the end of 1982.

There were three groups of patients. One group was treated only with antacids; the second group received similar antacids plus 150,000 i.u. of vitamin A; the third group were given the same doses of antacids and vitamin A as the second group but with the addition of the drug cyproheptadine.

All patients were treated for four weeks. Ulcer sizes were measured before and after treatment in each case.

Ulcers were all reduced to a significant degree, but the patients receiving vitamin A experienced a significantly greater reduction than those treated just with antacids. The authors concluded that 'a beneficial effect of vitamin A has been indicated in the prevention and treatment of stress ulcer in patients'.

Gastric ulcer can be thought of as a pre-cancerous state, and significant negative connection has been reported between low serum levels of vitamin A and the greater chance of development of lung, urinary, bladder and skin cancers. The results of this trial indicate a possible role for vitamin A in gastric protection by the prevention of the development of cancer from gastric ulcer!

Although the doses of vitamin A used are far beyond those acceptable for self-treatment, a daily supplementary intake of say 7,500 i.u. may be of benefit in those who have suffered from gastric and duodenal ulcers and wish to reduce the chances of others recurring. It may also help those with active ulcers to speed up their healing rate and protect them from further complications of their complaint.

Leg ulcers

VITAMIN E

Some leg ulcers are very resistant to conventional medical treatment and they often persist for long periods. They are prone to infection and cause a severe, burning and aching pain. Despite some 60 publications in medical journals on the effectiveness of vitamin E ointment for treating them, these ulcers are still a big problem for many people. They are associated with a poor blood supply to the limb, caused usually by varicose veins.

Application of the ointment and oral supplementation of the vitamin in the diet are usually sufficient to heal these ulcers. There is a word of caution from the proponents of this treatment, however. Once the ulcer has gone, oral supplementation of vitamin E should continue. This maintains local tissue oxygenation and blood circulation and prevents the ulcers from recurring.

Skin conditions, like acne and eczema, have responded to topical treatment with vitamin E ointment. There are many cases on record where multiple lacerations to the face as received in car accidents are completely and clearly healed up with combined topical and oral vitamin

E treatment. Many surgery units now use vitamin E ointment routinely after operations. It reduces toxic reactions, then soothes and heals the irritated area. A dose suitable for oral treatment is 400 i.u. vitamin E once daily, or two 250 i.u. capsules twice daily. This intake is perfectly safe when taken over the prolonged periods that may be needed, treating skin diseases as well as scars that have been left behind after accidents or surgery. A similar regime may help remove the stretch marks (striae) left behind after childbirth or some drug treatments.

Arthritis

PANTOTHENIC ACID

Young rats deprived of pantothenic acid developed joint inflammation and the hardening of their bones was impaired. Pigs and dogs were found to develop arthritic symptoms when pantothenic acid was missing from their diets.

A significant report then appeared in *The Lancet* regarding the blood pantothenic acid levels of various groups of people, with and without arthritis. What emerged was that the vegetarian group had significantly higher blood levels of pantothenic acid than those on a meat-eating diet.

The common factor in those suffering from arthritis, whether they were vegetarian or not, was the greatly reduced levels of pantothenic acid in their blood. In fact, the lower the level of pantothenic acid in the blood, the more severe were the symptoms of arthritis.

The two authors, Drs. E. C. Barton-Wright and W. A. Elliott then proceeded to test their hypothesis that rheumatoid arthritis is a vitamin-deficiency disease by treating arthritic patients with daily injections of 50mg calcium pantothenate. Within seven days, the blood levels of the vitamin increased and this was parallel by alleviation of the arthritic symptoms. This improvement persisted after further treatment for three weeks. However, discontinuing the supplementary calcium pantothenate caused the symptoms to return. Another report in the same journal from Dr. J. C. Annand claimed a similar result with the more difficult to treat serious disorder of osteo-arthritis.

These encouraging results led to a much larger trial of the vitamin in arthritis, organised by the General Practitioner Research Group and reported in *The Practitioner*. A total of 94 patients were involved and neither they nor the doctors knew whether the treatment was calcium pantothenate or a harmless placebo. Response to the treatment was assessed both by doctor and patient using a number of criteria. The dosage regime used was 500mg (1 tablet) daily for 2 days, 1,000mg (2 tablets) for 3 days, 1,500mg (3 tablets) for 4 days and finally 2,000mg (4 tablets) per day thereafter for a period of 2 months. Highly significant effects were recorded for calcium pantothenate in reducing the duration of morning stiffness, the degree of disability and the severity of pain.

Only in the condition of rheumatoid arthritis, however, was there any indication of a beneficial effect – there was little if any in the other types of arthritis. Why pantothenic acid should have this beneficial effect is not known with certainty, but an important clue lies in its function in controlling the synthesis of the anti-stress hormones of the body. Lack of the vitamin means lowered production of these hormones with subsequent development of inflammatory and degenerative diseases like arthritis. The ultimate treatment for these diseases consists of highly potent synthetic hormones known as corticosteroids. Pantothenic acid may enable the glands of the body to produce its own natural corticosteroids, so the end effect of either treatment is probably the same, but the vitamin therapy, of course, is far safer.

Reducing blood cholesterol

It is now generally believed that a high blood level of cholesterol increases the chances of fat deposition on the walls of blood vessels giving rise to the condition of atherosclerosis. The formation of a thrombus and hardening of the arteries (called arteriosclerosis) may also be more likely in those with high blood cholesterol levels. These high concentrations in the blood may also give rise to or be a consequence of excessive cholesterol in the bile which in turn predisposes to gall stone formation. Dietary measures to keep blood cholesterol in the normal range are now recommended as a general aid to good health. Vitamins taken at high doses may also contribute to control of cholesterol when this is high. What they will not do is reduce it below normal concentration.

NICOTINIC ACID

Nicotinic acid, but not nicotinamide, will reduce cholesterol levels in the blood. In a short term trial at the Mayo Clinic in the USA, 3g of nicotinic acid were given orally to patients with high blood cholesterol and levels were lowered to normal in 72 percent of those tested. The remaining 28 percent responded favourably to 4-6g per day. A longer term study over 11 years was carried out at the Dartmouth-Hitchcock Medical Centre in New Hampshire. A dose of 100mg nicotinic acid was given to 160 patients after each meal and this was increased over 11 days to 1g after each meal, at which level therapy continued. The average decrease in plasma cholesterol was 26 percent in those who took the vitamin for at least a year, and the lower cholesterol level was maintained for as long as treatment continued. It was particularly gratifying to note that there were no serious side-effects.

Other studies in Britain have indicated that nicotinic acid also has the property of lowering blood fats (triglycerides) in general at the above doses. In this respect it appears to be as effective as the drug clofibrate. It is believed to act in two ways; first, by inhibiting the synthesis of fats in the blood; and second, by competing with and preventing the release of free fatty acids which combine with cholesterol. These high potencies of nicotinic acid may not always be available so other means to reduce cholesterol may have to be sought. There is always the possibility too that this vitamin (but not nicotinamide) may cause transient flushing in some individuals. In either case, you may wish to control your blood cholesterol by other means.

VITAMIN C

Guinea-pigs, like man, require a dietary source of vitamin C and when deprived of the vitamin they show increased blood levels of cholesterol and fats are deposited in the walls of blood vessels of the heart and brain. They also show a greater tendency to produce gall-stones.

These and similar studies on human beings have been carried out by Dr. E. Ginter of Czechoslovakia. He found that diabetic patients (who usually have high blood cholesterol) and others with similar high levels responded to 500mg vitamin C daily.

The blood cholesterol level and the total fat in the blood were reduced in all cases. This reduction was maintained while those patients were given ample vitamin C. Similar supplementation on a group of patients who did not have high cholesterol levels had no effect. In other words, ascorbic acid will reduce excessive cholesterol, but once normal levels are achieved it has no further influence.

How does vitamin C achieve cholesterol reduction? It increases the rate at which cholesterol is converted into bile acids and hence excreted. In his patients Dr. Ginter found no evidence of a higher excretion of cholesterol as such, but what did increase dramatically was their excretion of bile acids. The usual route through which the body disposes of cholesterol is to convert it into bile acids in the liver, which are then deposited in the bile, carried to the intestine where they assist in fat digestion and end up excreted in the faeces. Speeding up this process disposes of excess cholesterol. Drugs that decrease cholesterol usually do so by preventing its synthesis by the body. Recently, however, these drugs have received adverse publicity because of their serious side-effects. It looks now as though we have in vitamin C a safe, effective treatment that works in a more logical manner, by accelerating the disposal of cholesterol. Blood fats are also reduced by vitamin C, but although the mechanism is not completely worked out, the vitamin is just as effective and safe.

In addition, there may be other benefits from an intake of 500mg of ascorbic acid daily. Dr. Geoffrey Taylor, formerly professor of medicine at the University of Lahore, has reported that changes in the tiny blood vessels, particularly those under the tongue, may be the warning signs of impending stroke. These changes also appear in scurvy and in mild deficiency of vitamin C. The number of deaths from strokes and coronary heart disease increases in cold weather in the winter, when the need for ascorbic acid is highest, but intake is at its lowest. Dr. Constance Lesley of the Wakefield Group of Hospitals in Yorkshire is another expert who has found that vitamin C exerts a powerful protective on certain high risk groups of the population. It may play a role in preventing heart attacks, strokes, deep vein thrombosis and atherosclerosis through its cholesterol and fat-controlling mechanisms. All of these conditions are less prevalent in vegetarians and this may reflect their higher dietary vitamin C intake.

VITAMIN E

We hear a lot of how high blood cholesterol levels can be a factor in the development of certain diseases but recent research suggests that total blood cholesterol is not the complete answer – we should also be looking at the types of cholesterol in the body. Cholesterol is carried on the backs of various proteins which are called VLDL (Very Low Density Lipoprotein); LDL (Low Density Lipoprotein); HDL (High Density Lipoprotein). The balance of these is important and when LDL and VLDL predominate, the chances of problems arising are increased. Therapy at reducing blood cholesterol is also additionally aimed at increasing the desirable HDL. Vitamin E appears to do just that.

Vitamin E can influence the cholesterol metabolism in two ways. First it has been shown that in some cases it can actually decrease cholesterol levels. Second, it can influence the proportion of the various lipoproteins in the blood in favour of the desirable HDL. In both functions, animal experiments using rabbits, which are partially susceptible in atherosclerosis, have confirmed the beneficial action of vitamin E.

A report in the *Journal of Nutrition* is typical. Rabbits were fed an athero-sclerosis-producing diet consisting of high butter intakes. There were three groups of animals on the diet; one group received supplementary vitamin E (the equivalent of a human adult receiving 400 i.u. daily); another group were fed BHA (butylated hydroxyanisole), a synthetic antioxidant much used in food and drugs; the third group were fed just the basic diet. After three years on the diets, there were significantly less frequent and less excessive atherosclerotic lesions in the aorta of those rabbits fed supplementary vitamin E than in the other two groups. Lower blood cholesterol levels were noted in the vitamin E group and it was this that was considered to be the main factor in inhibiting atherosclerosis.

Studies confirming that vitamin E can also reduce blood cholesterol levels in human beings were reported by Drs. M. Passeri and U. Butturini of the University of Parma, Italy in an International Symposium in Madrid. It was pointed out, however, that although this beneficial effect was related to a daily intake of 300 to 400 i.u. of vitamin E, extra vitamins A and C were more effective.

Other studies have indicated that 600 i.u. vitamin E taken for 30 days increased the proportion of HDL cholesterol from 9 percent to 40 percent. If the LDL cholesterol is high, the increase in HDL cholesterol is even more dramatic, up to 200 percent. In all cases blood-cholesterol levels were normal; vitamin E simply shifted the balance to the more desirable HDL cholesterol.

Respiratory infections

VITAMIN C AND THE COMMON COLD

Controversy over whether vitamin C taken in large doses can prevent or help relieve the symptoms of the common cold and other respiratory infections still rages but it now looks as if the trials confirming its benefits are outweighing those which were claimed to be negative. One reason is that daily intakes of the vitamins must be high to confer benefit; in many of the trials giving negative results they were carried out using relatively low doses.

Accordingly, a carefully controlled study with the relatively large amount of 1,000mg vitamin C was carried out by Dr. G. Ritzel of Switzerland. All of the 279 subjects were boys of similar age (16 to 17 years) and there were two periods of study, namely five and seven days. Neither investigators nor the boys knew whether they were taking their gram of ascorbic acid per day or a harmless placebo, so the trial was truly double-blind. The boys were examined daily by medical methods, for symptoms of colds and other infections and were also assessed on their own judgement symptoms. There was no doubt in this trial that vitamin C at the level given was of benefit in preventing and treating colds. Of the 140 subjects receiving placebo, 31 developed colds as against 17 out of 139 of those receiving 1,000mg of vitamin C. Moreover, the duration of the colds was some 29 percent less in the treated boys than those on placebo tablets.

A similar double-blind trial involving 641 children in a Navajo boarding school gave comparable results. Dr. J. L. Coulehan and his colleagues reported in the *New England Journal of Medicine* (1974), that giving 321 children 1g or 2g of ascorbic acid per day over 14 weeks reduced the average number of days with colds by 30 percent over a similar number of children not treated. They benefited in other ways too; in total there was 17 percent less time off sick, involving diseases other than those of the respiratory tract.

The most comprehensive and well-organised controlled trials were carried out in Toronto, Canada and reported in the *Canadian Medical*

Association Journal by Dr. T. W. Anderson and colleagues. The dosage regime varied slightly but the general conclusion was that 500 to 1,000mg vitamin C taken daily was a good preventative dose. If cold symptoms did develop, three grams per day was usually sufficient to reduce them. All subjects were assessed for their symptoms of respiratory disease and for their mental attitude. The investigators concluded that subjects in vitamin-treated groups experienced less severe illness than subjects not given vitamin C with approximately 25 percent fewer days spent indoors because of illness.

The longest and most successful clinical trial on record is that carried out by Dr. Edine Reginier of Massachusetts, USA, and report in the *Review of Allergy.* He treated 22 patients for five years, using the following regime: 600mg ascorbic acid at the first sign of a cold followed by 600mg every three hours, or 200mg every hour. At bedtime the amount taken was increased to 750mg. This quantity (4g per day) was continued for three or four days then reduced to 400mg every three hours for several days, further reducing to 200mg every three hours. With this regime, the vitamin C taken had bioflavonoids in addition, and of 34 colds, 31 were averted.

Excellent results were also obtained with vitamin C alone when 45 out of 50 colds were averted. This method of taking vitamin C at the onset of a cold is a sensible one and it avoids the sudden discontinuation of the vitamin that was a feature of less successful trials.

Mental Conditions

MILD DEPRESSION: PYRIDOXINE AND L-TRYPTOPHANE

A nerve substance called serotonin is produced constantly in the brain and at nerve endings. When it is not, serotonin levels drop and the results are a form of depression and sleep disturbance. The control of mood is dependent on brain concentrations of serotonin whose synthesis depends on two important food constituents, pyridoxine (vitamin B6) and the amino acid l-tryptophane. Lack of either of these will give similar symptoms to those when serotonin synthesis is reduced. Hence both or either may be used to overcome mild depression and to induce sleep.

We have seen already how a woman taking the contraceptive pill may develop mild depression because the constituents of the pill increase her requirements for vitamin B6. Similarly, even when not taking this form of contraception, a woman's needs for the vitamin can increase ten days or so before menstruation. In both cases the natural approach is to take 100mg daily of vitamin B6 for ten days before menstruation or to take 25 to 50mg of the vitamin daily from day ten of one cycle to day three of the next.

Sleep disturbances may be treated with the amino acid l-tryptophane if 500mg or 1,000mg of this is taken just before going to bed, but remember that this amino acid can only be prescribed by a medical practitioner. It is not recommended that greater doses of this should be taken, nor should the amino acid be taken during the day at this level since drowsiness may be induced. L-tryptophane at much higher doses can be prescribed for certain types of depression but this therapy should be under the supervision of a medical practitioner.

SCHIZOPHRENIA: NICOTINIC ACID AND NICOTINAMIDE

The mental symptoms associated with subclinical or mild pellagra are similar to those seen in schizophrenia and include tension, depression, personality problems and mental fatigue. These observations led Drs. H. Osmond and A. Hoffer of the University of Saskatchewan in Canada to suggest that this particular mental disease may respond to nicotinic acid in the same way as those who suffer from pellagra.

Accordingly, these doctors treated their first schizophrenic patients with high doses (3g to 6g) of the vitamin and reported dramatic results. They postulated that these patients had a biochemical abnormality that demanded a higher than usual intake of nicotinic acid so that even a good diet, supplying enough of the vitamin for the usual individual, was not sufficient. It was also suggested that a normal dietary intake of nicotinic acid could lead to a localized deficiency of the vitamin in the brains of these people. Although there was sufficient nicotinic acid to prevent the other symptoms of deficiency affecting the skin and digestive system it was believed that there was an abnormal barrier to the vitamin between the blood and brain in schizophrenia so that the brain was ostensibly starved of the vitamin.

Since these early successes, many doctors have reported similar results and clinics devoted to what is termed mega vitamin therapy have been founded. One such clinic is in New York where Dr. D. Hawkins has treated more than 4,000 patients with high doses of nicotinic acid. Where the acid cannot be tolerated at high levels, the neutral nicotinamide may be used. Sometimes better results were obtained when vitamin C was given at the same time. Doses of 4g each of nicotinic acid and vitamin C were required daily in some cases, with occasionally 50mg of vitamin B6. Dr. A. Cott reported in the journal *Schizophrenia* that it was also possible to administer high doses of these vitamins by injection in acute cases of the disease, but oral treatment could continue for several years.

No one should attempt self-treatment with these massive doses since each individual requires different amounts that depend upon personal requirements as well as upon any other treatments utilizing drugs. It must also be said there are clinical studies on record where no response was obtained when treating schizophrenics with nicotinic acid. Dr. C. C. Pfieffer, Chairman of the Brain Biocentre at Princeton, New Jersey believes that schizophrenic patients who have a high level of histamine in their bodies are less likely to respond to megadose nicotinic acid, and this may explain the varying responses to mega vitamin therapy.

Schizophrenic children may also respond to high doses of nicotinic acid or nicotinamide. Three grams of the vitamin, plus 500mg of vitamin B6 daily were reported by Dr. A. Hoffer to be of value in treating them and also hyperactive children. Those with poor learning ability often responded to 1-2g of nicotinic acid daily with the addition of the same amount of vitamin C, plus 200-400mg of vitamin B6. Dr. A. Cott believes that the reason for many of these mental diseases associated with childhood lies partly in an unbalanced diet high in refined foods plus an unusual demand for certain vitamins because of some biochemical abnormality. This is why they will respond only to doses far above those in the diet. Such doses can only be given under the supervision of a medical practitioner.

Mental Ability

THIAMINE

When we consider how essential thiamine is to nerve and brain function, it is perhaps not surprising that the vitamin appears to improve mental ability. In a study of children aged 9 to 19 years, Dr. R. F. Harvell of

Columbia University compared the effect of supplementation on one group, with the relatively low level of 2mg thiamine per day, with an unsupplemented group. Diets in both groups were identical and thought to be adequate. After one year there was a large increase in the mental achievements of those receiving the extra vitamin using the criteria of mental alertness, emotional stability, lack of depression and zest for life. Neither group at any time showed symptoms of B1 deficiency suggesting that the added vitamin was exerting an effect over and above that of the norm.

FOLIC ACID

A study from Masschusetts General Hospital, reported in the *New England Journal of Medicine* revealed that some mentally disturbed or retarded patients responded favourably to folic acid treatment. Even schizophrenics lose some of their psychotic symptoms. It has been mentioned previously that vitamin B6 is necessary in the production of certain chemicals that are normally released at nerve ending and folic acid too plays a part in the process. Certainly, in the above-mentioned study, it was found that both vitamin B6 and folic acid were essential in overcoming the mental symptoms. Neither was effective alone. Yet reports from Northwick Park Hospital, Middlesex have indicated that schizophrenia and other mental conditions have benefited from folic acid alone. What it agreed, however, is that some mental problems will respond to folic acid and at doses of only between 5mg and 20mg per day which must be taken under medical supervision.

VITAMIN B12

The knowledge that vitamin B12 deficiency produces nerve degeneration has stimulated studies into its use in brain and nerve disturbances. Old people with mild mental problems often respond to the vitamin. Dr. O. Abransky of the Hadassah University Medical School of Jerusalem has treated many old people who exhibited mental apathy, moodiness, poor memory, paranoia and confusion with vitamin B12 injections, bringing excellent results. A consultant psychiatrist at the University of Aberdeen, Dr. J. G. Handerson, has reported similar benefits in old people and believes that 'Vitamin B12 deficiency may be a possible diagnosis in the majority of psychiatric patients'. Mental disorders due to B12 deficiency are not confined to the old, and younger people often benefit from treatment with the vitamin. The fact that mental symptoms often appear before the anaemia associated with B12 deficiency would suggest that in these cases the patient's B12 level should be first examined. This is particularly so when an adequate intake of the vitamin from the food is in question.

CHOLINE

Choline, in the form of a simple derivative called acetylcholine, is essential in transmitting nerve impulses. Although nerves may be thought of as power cables - vehicles for carrying electric impulses – the resemblance ends where the nerve meets another nerve or the muscle it is controlling. Here electrical energy causes acetylcholine, which is stored in the nerve ending, to be released and in so doing it relays the message to the next nerve or to the muscle causing it to react. To prevent the acetylcholine from having a continuous action on the muscle, it is inactivated very quickly, allowing the muscle to relax and await the next nerve impulse, which starts the whole process over again. Lack of choline means that acetylcholine cannot be produced, so nerve function deteriorates with serious consequences. The therapeutic value of choline in this respect is seen in the treatment of senile dementia. Lecithin, which contains choline, has also been used.

A very recent development in the treatment of senile dementia is the use of choline as a simple dietary supplement in the form of lecithin. Experimental studies by Drs. M. J. Hirsch and R. J. Wurtman from the Massachusetts Institute of Technology showed that consumption of a single meal containing lecithin increased the levels of choline and its product acetylcholine in the brain of rats. Since acetylcholine is essential as a chemical transmitter in brain functioning, it seemed logical to try choline as a supplement in those conditions in man where acetylcholine may be deficient.

In a number of pilot studies this has been carried out on patients suffering from mental deterioration, with promising results. A typical trial was reported from Canada (*The Lancet*) when a dose of 25g of lecithin per day (i.e. 900mg choline) produced dramatic improvement in these patients. The treatment is a simple dietary one and is without side effects at the dose of 25g lecithin per day. What did emerge was that lecithin is preferable to choline as a food supplement. Choline is better absorbed as lecithin and there are more chances of side effects when choline itself is taken in high doses.

INOSITOL

This too is a constituent of lecithin, which may be regarded as its main dietary source. However, like choline, inositol and lecithin can be made by the body itself, although there do appear to be some conditions where body synthesis is insufficient. Dietary intakes and supplementation then assume importance. Supplementary doses may be as high as 1,000mg daily.

The brain and spinal cord nerves contain very high concentrations of inositol. Part of this is found in the myelin sheath, as with choline, but inositol appears to have some function not associated with its structural property. Thus Dr. C. C. Pfeiffer at the Brain Bio Centre, Princeton, New Jersey, USA, has studied the effect of inositol on brain wave patterns in schizophrenics and normal people. He claims that inositol has a similar anti-anxiety effect to that of the mild tranquilising drugs librium or meprobamate (e.g. Equagesic, Miltown). The calming effects of inositol can thus make it a possible alternative to the widely-prescribed librium and meprobamate. In this respect it is attractive to speculate that perhaps anxiety, irritability and hyperactivity may be related to a lack of inositol in the brain or some simple block in its metabolism.

All cells in the body appear to need inositol to stay healthy, but it is especially necessary for the bone marrow, eye membranes and the cells lining the gastro-intestinal tract. Unsubstantiated reports claim that it is food for stimulating good hair growth and the overcoming of baldness. These properties may be related to the role of inositol in maintaining cell structure in a healthy state.

High Blood Pressure and related conditions

Adequate intakes of all vitamins throughout life may prevent the onset of high blood pressure but, when taken at high dosage in supplementary form, some (vitamins C, E and the B vitamin choline in the form of lecithin) may also be used to treat the condition. Such natural approaches will in no way interfere with any medicinal drugs you may be taking for reducing high blood pressure and associated conditions – indeed they are almost certain to complement such drugs but they will not necessarily replace them. Always inform your practitioner if you are taking dietary or supplementary measures in addition to your medicinal drug therapy as it is possible that the latter may be reduced once the natural approach starts to benefit you.

Fat and cholesterol control

If fat and the associated cholesterol can be controlled and metabolised normally within the body, there are lessened chances of developing high blood pressure since this can be caused by the abnormal deposition of fats on the walls of blood vessels. As these vessels become constricted, the heart pumps harder and the pressure increases, to force blood through the narrowed orifice. Several vitamins function together to prevent the abnormal deposition of fats and these should in theory both prevent the condition of high blood pressure arising and hopefully to treat the preexisting condition.

LECITHIN

This is a complex fat composed of choline, inositol and polyunsaturated fatty acids (when obtained from soya), all of which contribute to its fat-fighting qualities.

Choline is defined as a lipotropic factor, which means that it prevents fats from accumulating in the liver by facilitating the transport of these fats to the organs that require them. Liver normally contains only between 5 and 7 percent of its weight as fat, but in the absence of choline this proportion can increase to as much as 50 percent. Such fatty deposits, when allowed to build up in the vital organ, adversely affect its normal functioning and the ill-effects are soon felt. There are a number of diseases that can give rise to fatty liver and these include diabetes, alcoholism and protein-deficiency. Lack of choline has been implicated in the development of fatty liver by Dr. S. Mookerjea of the University of Toronto, who observed an increase of liver fats during periods of choline deprivation.

When fats are transported from the liver, they do so in the form of complex substances called phospholipids. These are composed of fats, phosphorus, sugar and choline in combination. According to experimental evidence from animal work published in the *American Journal of Clinical Nutrition*, lack of choline prevented this mechanism from operating with the result that the liver cells soon filled up with unwanted fat. Supplementation with choline not only prevented such changes but actually reserved the process and cleared the liver of accumulated fat. Human studies on infants suffering from fatty liver (*Journal of the American Medical Association*) have confirmed a similar role for choline in human beings.

It is possible that prolonged low levels of choline in the body can give rise to high blood pressure (hypertension). The compound was given to a group of patients suffering from hypertension with beneficial results according to a report in the *Journal of Vitaminology*. Typical symptoms of palpitations, dizziness and headaches disappeared within two weeks of treatment, together with reduction of the blood pressure to normal. The mechanism of this action is not known, but it could be via the nerves by controlling the blood vessels, which in turn determine the blood pressure. Other evidence suggests that low levels of choline throughout life may put some individuals on the road to hypertension in later years.

INOSITOL

We have seen above how important choline is as a lipotropic agent in ensuring that fat is kept in solution and is not deposited in the wrong places in the body. The second factor that also has this property is inositol, but it is structurally very different from choline and hence exerts its lipotropic action in a different way. The fat-fighting properties of inositol appear to act in addition to those associated with choline, so it is not surprising that both are essential in controlling fat metabolism. There are reports from the *American Heart Journal* by Drs. I. Leinwand and D. H. Moore that giving 3g of inositol daily to atherosclerotic patients resulted in a reduction of blood fats and cholesterol. Similar treatment reduced the excessive depositions of fat in those suffering from fatty liver. Despite these early reports, however, it is now accepted that the best way to restore fat metabolism to normal is by treating with both choline and inositol. Drs. D. A. Sherber and M. M. Levites reported in the *Journal of The American Medical Association* that this approach was successful in reducing cholesterol levels in all their patients subjected to the treatment.

Adequate intakes of both choline and inositol, along with polyunsaturated fatty acids, can be obtained by taking 15 to 30 grams of lecithin daily in the form of granules. Along with other measures, this can usefully be employed to treating high blood pressure and heart conditions.

Circulatory Problems

VITAMIN E

The main groups of diseases that have responded to vitamin E are essentially those of the blood circulating system, where for one reason or another, the flow of blood to an organ or muscle has been curtailed. This may be due to a blood clot (thrombosis); a narrowing of the blood vessel due to deposition of fat (atherosclerosis); a hardening of the artery (arteriosclerosis); a swollen and knotted condition of the veins (varicose veins); blood clots in the veins (thrombophlebitis).

Other conditions include high blood-pressure, heart failure, sterility, menstrual problems and ageing. In addition, some skin diseases – including severe ulceration – have been reported to respond to vitamin E treatment.

Intermittent Claudication

This is the term that describes the cramping pain in the calf muscles that is produced on exercise. It is caused by a narrowing of the arteries supplying blood to the leg muscles. The restricted blood supply gives rise to the pain as the muscles become starved of oxygen. A leading article in *The Lancet* states that this is the only generally accepted use of vitamin E in medical practice. Dr. P. D. Livingstone and Dr. C. Jones reported the results of a double-blind clinical trial of vitamin E in intermittent claudication carried out at Sheffield.

Out of 17 patients who were treated with 600 i.u. of d-alpha tocopherol per day for a total period of 40 weeks, 13 showed significant improvement in their ability to walk without pain. Only 2 of the 17 patients treated with the placebo reported some improvement over a similar period. It was essential to continue treatment for at least 3 months before any improvement became apparent. It was also noted that the vitamin E-treated patients had an increased life survival rate. Eventually this research group was able to report some years later that some 1,500 patients suffering from intermittent claudication had responded favourably and significantly to tocopherol treatment.

Angina Pectoris

Angina pectoris is a condition characterized by a severe, constricting pain in the chest, usually radiating to one or both arms and shoulders. The pain is due to a temporary insufficiency of blood to the heart that deprives the heart muscle of oxygen. It is a similar situation to the one in intermittent claudication, except that the heart muscle itself is affected instead of the legs. In both cases the attack is relieved by rest.

According to the Shute Institute, where many thousands of angina patients have been treated with vitamin E, the angina condition usually responds in four to six weeks from the start of the treatment. The initial dose is usually 800 i.e. d-alpha tocopherol per day. If there is no improvement after six weeks on this dose, the daily intake is increased by 200 to 400 i.e. for the next six weeks.

When the dose at which the symptoms are relieved is reached, this is continued permanently. Such doses apply only when the blood pressure is controlled by drugs. Even if there is not complete relief with this treatment, it is important for anyone suffering from angina to take d-alpha tocopherol to prevent blood clots or thrombosis from forming.

Coronary Heart Disease

D-alpha tocopherol helps in coronary heart disease by:

1. Dissolving the blood clot that is causing the obstruction.

2. Decreasing the oxygen needs of the whole zone of injury, so preserving its structure and function.

3. Dilating the blood vessels, so allowing more blood and hence more oxygen to reach the damaged portion of the heart. Continuous use of tocopherol following a heart attack prevents further occurrence of a blockage. Although the heart muscle that has died (known as an infarct) can never be restored, vitamin E treatment ensures that the surrounding area receives adequate oxygen and helps restore it to health.

Even when vitamin E therapy is started immediately after the heart attack, it may take a week or 10 days before any benefit is felt. A study was carried out on 22 patients by Dr. W. M. Toone and reported in the *New Zealand Journal of Medicine*. Eleven of his patients received 1,600 i.u. of d-alpha tocopherol succinate per day after their heart attacks, while the remaining eleven received a placebo. Seven of the treated patients were able to eliminate conventional medical treatment, and all felt the benefit of vitamin E. Only three of the control group were able to reduce this medical treatment.

Other studies at the Shute Institute on many hundreds of patients have indicated an overall success rate of 60 percent of patients receiving vitamin E after a heart attack. The usual procedure is to start such patients on 800 i.u. of vitamin E per day and increase this by 200 i.u. increments every six weeks until a response is obtained. Once the dosage is established, the individual keeps it at that level for the rest of his life.

Arteriosclerosis and Cerebral Thrombosis

A similar dosage regime is carried out on those whose heart blood vessels are constricted by hardening, a condition usually associated with ageing. When a similar condition affects the brain blood vessels, the usual symptoms are forgetfulness, lack of concentration and impaired mental ability in the aged. In both cases vitamin E may be helpful but the addition of vitamin C at a dose of 2g to 5g per day is now known to be particularly beneficial.

A constriction of the blood supply to the brain (called cerebral thrombosis) may give rise to a stroke resulting in temporary or permanent paralysis of part of the body. Treatment with vitamin E is essentially the same as that when the heart is similarly affected. Not only does vitamin E help dissolve the obstruction but it prevents further development of a thrombosis.

Varicose Veins

Another disease of the blood circulatory system is varicose veins. The conventional medical treatment for this condition is surgery. This may be avoided in some cases by treating with vitamin E but the dosage varies over a wide range. Dr. W. Shute in his book Vitamin E for Ailing and Healthy Hearts quotes many successful treatments of varicose veins with vitamin E.

The dose usually begins at 150 i.u. or 300 i.u. per day which is increased in increments of 100 i.u. every six weeks if no improvement is noted. Most people respond to 300 or 600 i.u. but some need the high dose of 800 i.u. per day before relief is obtained. One of the complications of varicose veins can be the development of ulcers (called indolent ulcers), that are very resistant to healing. Oral vitamin E has been claimed to cut down the incidence of these.

Menstrual and Menopausal problems

There are many reports of the beneficial effects of vitamin E in relieving the painful periods suffered by some women and in normalizing the cycle where this is irregular. Heavy and scanty menstrual flows are not influenced by the vitamin.

According to the Shute Institute, vitamin E exerts its action in women by normalizing the blood levels of the female sex hormones, known as oestrogens. It dilates the blood vessels, so ensuring a good supply of blood to the womb. At the same time, the vitamin improves the heat–regulating capacity of the body, which is why it helps in excessive sweating that is often a feature of the menopause.

Menstrual abnormalities are often treated with oestrogen. However, many obstetricians and gynaecologists who have used vitamin E believe it is safer to let the vitamin stimulate the body's own production of oestrogens. There is a certain risk in treating women with sex hormones, particularly during the menopause, when their production starts to slow down. By treatment with vitamin E, it is believed that the transition to decreased production of oestrogens, with its accompanying effects, is smoother and easier. Similarly, irregular oestrogen synthesis which can give rise to problems in younger women may be normalized by vitamin E treatment.

The use of vitamin E in the menopause has been actively studied by Dr. Henry A. Gozan of New York. In the *New York State Journal of Medicine* he reported that treatment with vitamin E helped relieve the flushing, headaches and nervous symptoms associated with the menopause. There was success in easing and eliminating these distressing symptoms in 59 out of 66 patients so treated. The dosage used was 100 i.u. of the vitamin taken three times daily over a three month period.

Sunburnt and Scalded Skin

Many medical papers testify to the effectiveness of vitamin E in the form of cream or ointment in treating damaged skin, whether caused by burns, sunburn or scalding liquids. No matter what the agent is, treatment consists of covering the affected area as quickly as possible with a cream or ointment containing from 30 to 100 i.u. of vitamin E per gram. Typical treatments have been described by Dr. Wilfred E. Shute in his book *Vitamin E for Ailing and Healthy Hearts*. The time to respond varies from hours in the case of simple sunburn, to weeks when the skin is badly scalded but the important result is a minimum or complete lack of scarring.

A boy of six was scalded badly with multiple burns over his neck, torso, back, chest and thigh. An attempt at skin-grafting was not only unsuccessful but left whole areas of raw flesh that were badly infected. This persisted for 10 weeks. Treatment with vitamin E was then initiated. After 10 days, the infection was cleared but the damaged areas remained very raw and painful. Application of vitamin E ointment was continued, along with a daily oral dose to 300 i.u. Complete healing occurred after 13 weeks. What was particularly gratifying was to find that the scars were smooth, painless and contracted into weals. Skin-grafting was not even needed.

Older people respond just as dramatically. A woman aged 58 received scalds over a wide area of her torso and the damage was worsened by leaving on her clothing, which retained the hot water next to the skin. Conventional medical treatment with brine baths failed, leaving her with a grossly infected skin. Treatment was switched to oral and topical vitamin E. Within five days healing commenced and continuation of the treatment for three months resulted in complete cure.

Dr. Wilfred E. Shute attributes the healing properties of vitamin E on the skin to three unique characteristics:

1. It lessens or removes the associated pain a few minutes after application.

2. It stops the burn from deepening, limiting the damage to the cells actually destroyed by the burning agent.

3. It stimulates rapid regeneration of new skin, giving a scar that is not painful, is of the same height as surrounding skin and is not contracted.

The mild antiseptic quality of vitamin E may help against infection but other measures are usually needed to keep the affected area clean. Once this is controlled, the healing action of the vitamin is both quick and effective.

Other conditions that may respond to Vitamin Therapy

Kidney Stones

The most common kind of kidney stones are formed from an insoluble mineral called calcium oxalate. This is composed of calcium and oxalic acid, both normal constituents of food. In addition, oxalic acid is produced by the body during its normal metabolic processes. Yet some people form stones and others do not, despite having similar diets. The ability to form stones depends upon two factors; first how well the calcium oxalate can be kept in solution; and second, the control of oxalic acid production. The first factor depends upon the presence of adequate magnesium since the ratio of calcium to magnesium determines the solubility of calcium oxalate. The second factor is related to vitamin B6, since when this is deficient there is an increase in oxalic acid production. Adequate pyridoxine protects by reducing the formation of this potential precipitating agent.

These observations were put to the test in a clinical study carried out at Harvard University by Drs. E. L. Prienard and S. N. Gershoff and reported in the *American Journal of Clinical Nutrition*. A total of 265 patients with histories of chronic kidney stone formation were treated with 240mg magnesium and 20mg of vitamin B6 per day. A staggering 89 percent of these patients benefited from the course of supplementation. They stopped producing kidney stones and remained free of them while on the mineral/vitamin treatment. This simple treatment is safe and effective, but it is preferably taken in conjunction with a calcium-controlled diet, a regime that kidney stone sufferers are already familiar with.

Bronchial Asthma

Vitamin B6 has been referred to as the anti-allergy vitamin, mainly on account of its successful use in some allergic skin diseases, in hay fever and in bronchial asthma. Comprehensive studies by a team of doctors at Nassau County Medical Centre, USA, headed by Dr. P. J. Collipp have indicated that pyridoxine is remarkably safe and effective treatment for some asthma sulferers. The clue to the treatment was provided by the observation that many asthma victims show abnormal metabolism of vitamin B6 when tested with the tryptophan loading test. Consequently, in one trial, 38 asthmatic children received 100mg of vitamin B6, twice per day and a similar number received a harmless placebo. Neither patients nor doctors knew what they were given – in fact this was a true double-blind study. The effect of the treatment was assessed by noting such criteria as wheezing, difficult breathing, cough, tightness in the chest and outright asthmatic attacks.

Only starting with the second month did those receiving vitamin B6 show any definite clinical improvement over those receiving placebo. From then on, however, the improvement was maintained in every aspect of the disease. No side-effects were observed during the five-month duration of the trial. It must be stressed that existing drug treatment of the individuals continued, but as this was palliative rather than curative, (e.g. the use of bronchodilators), it was gradually phased out under medical guidance. The researchers could not explain why the vitamin has this beneficial effect, but they admit that pyridoxine appears to be acting as a drug rather than as a vitamin. It is possible that the children are suffering from a B6-dependency, so that for some reason their requirements for the vitamin are particularly high and cannot be obtained simply from the diet. Adult sufferers from asthma also benefit from a similar dosage but the positive response to the vitamin is not outstanding as that in children. These beneficial doses of vitamin B6 should only be taken under supervision of a qualified practitioner.

Insect bites

Those who suffer from the excessive attentions of insects can be helped by vitamin BI according to a report in *Medical Letters* and subsequent reports. Out of 100 sufferers in one trial, more than 70 percent reported that on an intake of 75 to 100mg daily, insects bothered them little or not at all. It is highly unlikely that at this level of intake the thiamine is acting in its true vitamin role, but rather as a therapeutic internal insect repellent. No side-effects were noted in this trial. This protective effect has not been noted in everyone probably because some people may require even higher intakes of the vitamin. It does appear likely though that the vitamin functions by finding its way to the skin where its odour, detectable bv insects but not by human beings, may act as a deterrent.

Carpal Tunnel Syndrome

Carpal tunnel syndrome is due to a compression of the median nerve as it enters the palm of the hand. This causes pain and numbness in the index and middle fingers and weakness of the muscle of the thumb. The condition is relatively common and can affect either one or both hands. Women are most affected and the syndrome is often seen during the last third period of pregnancy. Vitamin B6 has been found to relieve the condition. The usual dose is 50mg of the vitamin daily during the first three months of pregnancy and this is usually sufficient to prevent the syndrome in the last three months. Vitamin B6 at this level must not be taken by a pregnant woman without the knowledge of her doctor. In other people, 50-250mg of vitamin B6 daily may be needed to relieve the pain of the syndrome and the dose must be continued for at least 12 weeks. Stiffness in the fingers of diabetics will often be relieved by vitamin B6 at daily doses between 50 and 100mg. The problem in diabetic children may be overcome by daily doses of 25mg of the vitamin.

Food allergies and supplementation

Foods may provoke a wide variety of allergic symptoms by multiple mechanisms but the release of histamine is one of the most important. Histamine is found in nearly all of the tissues of the body but is associated mainly with mast cells. During inflammation and allergic response, mast cells release a variety of chemicals amongst which is histamine which has pronounced pharmacological activity that serves to protect the body. However, when the histamine is released under abnormal stimulus such as allergens in food, the responsive mechanisms can cause undesirable symptoms. Hence the development of anti-histamines that neutralise the effect of the released substance.

It has been established that when blood vitamin C levels are low, blood histamine levels are high. Giving supplemental vitamin C causes reduction of these high histamine concentrations. This was observed in 1981 when 437 normal subjects deliberately reduced their blood levels of vitamin C by withdrawing it from their diets. As the levels of vitamin decreased so whole blood histamine levels increased. Once ascorbate concentration dropped below 0.7mg per 100ml blood, the increase in blood histamine levels was highly significant. In another study, when vitamin C blood levels were low or histamine blood levels were high, a daily dose of one gram of the vitamin restored histamine levels to normal in only 3 days. The same amount of the vitamin given along with 10mg vitamin BI reduced the symptoms of allergic rhinitis substantially in 75% of the people affected.

The fat soluble vitamin E also is regarded as an antihistamine vitamin. Volunteers who had severe swelling at the site after injection of histamine had a much reduced response when pretreated with 400 i.u. vitamin E for 5-7 days. Vitamin B12 is a water-soluble vitamin that has exhibited anti-histamine activity in conditions of intractable asthma, chronic urticaria and allergic dermatitis – all conditions that can be induced by food ingredients. However, the vitamin must be in a high potency injection into the muscle (1000μg) since because of limited absorption, oral tablets will not give high enough body levels.

Monosodium glutamate (MSG) widely used in food preparation as a flavour enhancer is also one of the most common allergens in the diet. Taking vitamin C before food containing MSG will protect adverse allergic effects of the flavour enhancer which can be very distressing to some people causing serious flushing, headaches, dizziness and nerve problems. MSG sensitivity can also be controlled by vitamin B6. In an experimental double-blind study reported in 1981, a daily dose of 50mg vitamin B6 was given to 9 students who had exhibited strong allergic response to MSG previously while 3 researchers received placebo. After 12 weeks therapy with the vitamin those who suffered from MSG no longer did so and those on placebo continued to respond to it.

Bioflavonoids, notably catechin and quercetin, are found in all diets but are particularly rich in fruits and vegetables. Like vitamin C, which they invariably accompany in the food, bioflavonoids are excellent oral anti-histamines. Catechin for example functions in two ways. First, it inhibits the release of histamine from the mast cells and second, it inhibits the enzyme needed to convert the amino acid histidine into histamine. This conversion is a continuous process in the mast cells. Catechin has been given to people with food allergies and as long as it was given before the allergenic food, it prevented an allergic response. Quercetin, another bioflavonoid in our food, acts in a similar manner and its effect in the pure state is so great that it has been used to suppress the symptoms of allergic asthma. Although our diet provides both allergenic substances and anti-allergen constituents, the balance is usually in favour of the former which is why some people will continue to respond adversely to these undesirable substances. Fortunately, other food constituents like the vitamins and bioflavonoids when taken in amounts far beyond those found in the diet can help neutralise the effects of allergenic food substances.

Drug addiction

Addictive drugs can adversely affect nutritional status in the same way as alcoholism does so the supplementary approach to reduce the ravages of body organs by these alien substances is similar. As the liver, followed closely by the kidneys, is the organ most targetted by addictive drugs, it is essential to maintain levels of the antioxidant vitamins plus the whole of the vitamin B complex. A high potency vitamin B complex preparation providing 25 to 50mg of B1, B2, niacin, pyridoxine, and pantothenic acid plus 400µg of folic acid, 100µg biotin and 100µg vitamin B12 should be taken on a daily basis. Typical antioxidant intakes are vitamin C 1000mg daily; vitamin E 400 i.u. daily; beta-carotene 15mg daily; vitamin A 7500 i.u. daily; coenzyme Q10, 30mg three times daily. An amino acid supplement containing all of the essential amino acids as the preferred substances can help restore liver and kidney function – as can the essential fatty acids (omega-3 zinc (15mg) and selenium (200µg) taken daily are also essential, and omega-6 types) which are depleted in drug addition. All of these dietary nutrients can help in two ways: first they ensure that the detoxification of the drugs is at maximum efficacy and second, they restore normal levels to the vital organs affected. Thus this nutritional approach can [1] prevent or reverse the damage done by addictive drugs [2] perhaps reduce the craving for drugs (proved in animal experiments but not yet in human beings) [3] reduce the symptoms of drug withdrawal. Supplementation is not sufficient on its own. It must be accompanied by a properly supervised drug withdrawal programme. Benefits are best felt after total withdrawal of drugs.

How safe are Vitamins?

As far as self-help with supplementary vitamins is concerned only two of them, A and D, should be regarded as likely to give rise to toxic side-effects when taken in very high doses. For this reason the UK authorities have suggested, and indeed in some cases have legislated for, a maximum supplementary daily intake of vitamin A of 7,500 i.u. (2.25mg). In the case of vitamin D, no more than 400 i.u. (10µg), should be taken on a daily basis. On prescription of course, and hence under medical supervision, higher potencies can be obtained and taken.

The limits above apply only to products containing vitamins A and D that are available on general sale and the golden rule is – take these supplements only at the daily dose recommended on the pack. There is no point in anyone in this country and in the Western world in general taking more than 7,500 i.u. vitamin A and 400 i.u. vitamin D on a regular basis. Remember that these vitamins are being taken in addition to those in the diet and the supplementary limits take dietary intakes into account. Dosing yourself with more than the recommended amount will do no more good than taking that suggested on the pack. If you feel you need much higher intakes of vitamin A and D for one reason or another then you obviously need professional medical advice.

To these two fat-soluble vitamins must now be added a water-soluble one, pyridoxine or vitamin B6. Some side-effects have been reported in people taking massive doses of pyridoxine on a daily basis over many months. Most of these individuals were taking between 2,000 and

6,000mg of the vitamin daily. One case of side-effects in a person taking 500mg daily for a long period has also been reported but this response should be regarded as most unusual.

When we look at these reports in perspective they can be seen as representing quite abnormal and unnecessary potencies of the vitamin. Daily intakes below these have not been reported as causing any ill-effects in the many trials where pyridoxine has been taken to treat premenstrual syndrome or the side-effects of the contraceptive pill. It would need for example, 20 of the highest potency vitamin B6 preparations (100mg) available in the UK, taken daily for many months, to allow the lower toxicity level of 2,000mg to be reached. Much higher potencies are available in the USA which probably explains why this is where toxicity problems were reported.

Self-help with all vitamins can be beneficial to many people but remember to take only the dosage recommended on the pack unless higher intakes are suggested by a medical or other practitioner.

Safe intakes of vitamins fall into two categories: those for long-term consumption and those for short-term consumption. In both cases the figures refer to the total intake from all food sources plus supplementary amounts and not from supplementation alone. Short-term consumption should be regarded as daily intakes for three months or less. When no limit has been established for short-term consumption, the figures quoted for long term consumption may be regarded as a safe intake over an indefinite period. The following table sums up upper safe levels and upper limits. All figures are taken from publications by the *European Federation of Health Product Manufacturers Association* (EHPM) 1997.

SAFE INTAKES OF VITAMINS

Nutrient	Unit	Upper Safe Level Long Term Consumption	Upper Limit Short Term Consumption
Vitamin A (retinol equiv)	µg	3000	7500
In pregnancy	µg	800	800
Vitamin D	µg	20	50
Vitamin E (as d-alpha toxopherol equiv)	mg	800	None established
B-Carotene	mg	25	None established
Thiamin	mg	50	None established
Riboflavin	mg	200	None established
Nicotinamide	mg	1500	3000
Nicotanic acid	mg	500	1000
Nicotinic acid – slow release	mg	250	500
Pyridoxine	mg	200	200
Folic acid	µg	1000	None established
Vitamin B12	µg	3000	None established
Biotin	µg	2500	None established
Pantothenic acid	mg	1000	None established
Vitamin C	mg	1000	None established

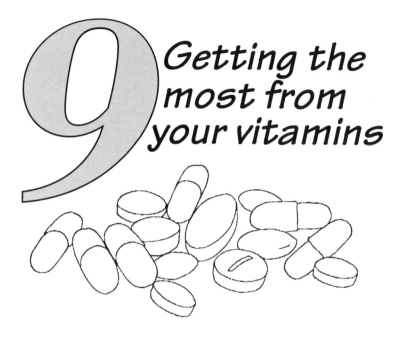

9 Getting the most from your vitamins

Despite the ever-growing number of people who feel the need to take extra vitamins in tablet or soft-gelatine capsule form, there is no doubt that our basic needs for these micronutrients should be from the daily diet. Adequate daily requirements of vitamins can be met solely from the food, on the assumption that this is freshly picked, cooked expertly with an eye to preserving the vitamins, and eaten as soon as possible after preparations. Such considerations are fine in theory but often impossible to achieve in practice, yet a few simple rules will ensure that you are getting the most from the vitamins in your diet.

The vitamin B complex and vitamin C are all water-soluble so that when boiling food, more losses are due to leaching into the water than simple destruction. As long as the water is then used in the preparation of a sauce or gravy the leached vitamins are retrieved and contribute an important proportion of the day's requirements. Short term boiling in a minimum amount of water retains far more vitamins in all vegetables than long term boiling in a lot of water. However, the steaming and pressure cooking of green vegetables is to be preferred to boiling, although the difference in vitamins leached from root vegetables is not as great when cooking losses for these three methods are compared.

Deep freezing of foods represents a good way of preserving vitamins but the process is preceded by blanching which itself can cause some preliminary loss. Microwave blanching causes less damage to vitamin levels than hot water treatment because of the leaching losses referred to overleaf. Don't forget though that the act of thawing allows vitamins to escape into the thawed water. This is of less importance in frozen vegetables which can be cooked immediately from the frozen state but losses can be significant in meats and poultry where thawing periods of up to 24 hours are usually recommended before cooking commences. Utilizing the thawed liquors will help you recapture those vitamins that got away. Losses by leaching of boiled frozen vegetables are just as large as those when fresh vegetables are boiled, sometimes they are greater since the acts of freezing and thawing ruptures cells, allowing more of the contents to escape.

Studies on the preservatives of vitamins during microwave cooking have given variable results. For example vitamin C is better retained in broccoli, cabbage and carrots after microwave cooking than after boiling, but shows little difference to pressure cooking. In potatoes, pressure cooking and boiling are far superior to microwave cooking in respect of vitamin C retention so it is not possible to draw hard and fast rules. Nevertheless, on the whole, microwave cooking can be regarded as a satisfactory process as far as the preservation of water-soluble vitamins is concerned.

Fat-soluble vitamins pose less problems when it comes to consideration of losses during boiling and its associated processes. Vitamin A, carotene and vitamin D are all relatively stable because of their water insolubility. Light should be regarded as the main destroyer of vitamin A. Along with vitamin E these fat soluble vitamins are susceptible mainly to oxidizing agents so vitamin C, which tends to accompany these vitamins in foods, affords the best protection against oxygen during food processing. Vitamin E is unique in being unstable during frozen storage, so you should not assume that it is available to you if you have a high intake of frozen foods.

Let us see how vitamins are presented in food and how they are dealt with by the digestive system because then it is possible to glean much information about the best way to make use of them. In a typical meal the vitamins are an integral part of the food constituents and are often present attached to fats or proteins. Usually, therefore, as the food is digested the vitamins are liberated and become available for absorption. Digestion is a slow process so not all the vitamins are released at one time – it is more a case of gradual leaching of them into the gastro-intestinal tract. With the exception of B12, vitamins are generally absorbed over quite a length of the digestive tract so that assimilation also happens over a number of hours. This is the situation in food, but what happens when a vitamin tablet or capsule is swallowed?

First, the rate of release of the vitamin depends on the time of disintegration of the tablet or that of dissolution of the gelatine shell of the capsule. In any preparation (apart from the prolonged release variety) this should be between 15 and 30 minutes, which means that all of the vitamin becomes available for absorption at one time. When absorption of the vitamin is an active process via specific sites in the digestive tract, such sites become saturated very quickly. The result is that some of the vitamin is passed on without being absorbed. When the vitmin is absorbed by simple diffusion, these considerations do not apply and assimilation is more efficient. Sometimes, of course, a rapid, high level of a particular vitamin in the blood is required, as for example in treating respiratory virus infections with vitamin C, but the more natural supplementation calls for a steady maintenance of adequate blood levels of the vitamin.

Hence, if we wish to mimic nature in the provision of vitamins to the body, tablets or capsules taken with each meal is one aproach but, nevertheless, these micronutrients are still released too quickly. A better approach is to simulate what happens in the course of digestion of a normal meal and this can only be achieved by taking an effective prolonged (or sustained) release formulation. A good product will release its vitamin steadily at an even rate over the necessary 6, 8 and 12-hour period in exactly the way they would be if present in food. These, too, are best taken with food because then the ingredients of the tablet or capsule will move along the digestive tract at the same rate as the food it accompanies.

One of the more controversial subjects in vitamin supplementation is whether naturally-derived vitamins offer advantages over the synthetic variety. If we look at the evidence available there is little doubt that the scales come down in favour of the natural vitamins. We get more out of these for the following reasons. Most vitamins can exist in two forms, which for convenience we can refer to as right-handed (d) and left-handed (l). This is simply a quirk of their chemical structure and the difference may appear to be minimal when viewed in a chemical light. Nevertheless, in terms of biological activity, the body is very selective and it can use only one of the forms, the other being virtually useless. Not surprisingly, in foods and other natural sources, nature provides the correct biological form of the vitamin. Sometimes it is the d-form, other times the l-form, there are no hard and fast rules, but the natural form represents that most efficiently used by the body. A prime example is d-alpha tocopherol, the natural form of vitamin E, which on a milligram for milligram basis is 49 percent more active than the synthetic dl variety. Nature is rather more clever than the chemist when it comes to making vitamin E. Whereas in nature the d-form alone is produced, the chemist can only make the dl-form, i.e. 50 percent of each type. It is possible for the chemist to resolve his dl-vitamin E and isolate just the d-form but his yield is only 50 percent and the l-form is wasted. It is just not worth the expense to separate the two types so the chemist offers the mixture and allows the body to select the form of vitamin E it can use.

Although d-alpha tocopherol is regarded as the natural form of vitamin E, it does not occur in nature on its own. Food sources of the vitamin invariably contain a mixture of four different types called d-alpha, d-beta, d-gamma and d-delta-tocopherols. In most biological test systems the most active vitamin E on a milligram for milligram basis is d-alpha tocopherol. However, in terms of anti-oxidant activity, which represents possibly the most important protective function of vitamin E, d-delta tocopherol is the most potent. Such differences reflect the wisdom of ensuring an intake, dietary or supplementary, of all the tocopherols since it could be wrong to assess the activity of the whole group simply on one criterion or another.

Vitamin C (ascorbic acid) appears rather easier to deal with because this is one case where the chemist can synthesize in the laboratory exactly the type of the vitamin that occurs in nature, namely l-ascorbic acid. Hence it is well-nigh impossible for anyone to detect the difference between vitamin C isolated from the acerola cherry and that produced in a laboratory because they are both the l-form. Nevertheless, there are differences in the way the body can use the vitamin C present in acerola powder and that present as pure ascorbic acid. The secret lies in the substances that accompany the vitamin in the natural source that are not present in the synthetic variety.

These substances are the bioflavonoids which are always associated with vitamin C when it occurs naturally. The body, too, appears to require them for the most efficient utilization of vitamin C in some of its functions. As the bioflavonoids (sometimes called vitamin P) and ascorbic acid function together in the maintenance of the health and integrity of the blood vessels it is sensible to take both together in tablets or capsules as they are taken thus in the diet.

The example of vitamin C and the bioflavonoids illustrates neatly the prime difference between naturally occurring and synthetic vitamins. The former are superior in their biological action because they are presented in their natural environment. This means that even in tablet or capsule form, vitamin C is best utilized when it is accompanied by rose hip powder, acerola cherry powder or some other natural source of the vitamin and the bioflavonoids. The B vitamins are more efficiently assimilated in the presence of yeast or liver powder. Vitamin E is preferred in the oil from which it is derived, be it wheat germ or soya.

Not only are such preparations presenting the vitamins in the environment that nature supplies them in but there is always the possibility that the accompanying substances confer greater activity on the vitamin (as with vitamin C and the bioflavonoids). Yeast is a complex organism containing all the B vitamins, apart from vitamin B 12, but it is possible that there are also present some, as yet, unknown factors that need to accompany the vitamins we already know about. There could even be more unidentified vitamins present that you can obtain only from natural sources.

There is, however, one vitamin that is probably utilized better from tablets than from the food itself. This is folic acid, which in the natural form exists both as the free acid and as the acid conjugated or combined with glutamic acid residues of up to six in number. Free folic acid is far better absorbed than conjugated folic acid. Hence if a food supplies mainly the conjugated variety not much of it will actually be assimilated by the body. Peanuts for example contain in 100g only 28μg of free folic acid, but 82μg of the conjugated form which is less readily absorbed. On the other hand, 100 gram of cabbage yields 60μg of the free form along with only 30μg of the conjugated acid, which means that most of the vitamin is readily absorbed. In tablet form, folic acid is usually presented as the free acid so we would expect a higher efficiency of absorption.

It has often been said the vitamin of the B complex are better utilized when all are presented in the same formulation in the correct balance as that found in foods. This is true up to a point as for example in the situation, not uncommon, where there is a mild deficiency of the B vitamins across the whole spectrum. A poor diet or a stress situation is more likely to cause a mild deficiency of the whole complex so it is not unreasonable to supplement with all of them. Situations do arise, however, where a particular deficiency is induced usually by treatment with a specific medicinal drug. The contraceptive pill, for example, is notorious in increasing the requirements of vitamin B6 in the female. Taking it and this vitamin alone, in potencies of 50mg upwards, is often sufficient to overcome the mild depression associated with this form of contraception. In such cases because the synthetic hormones are inducing a specific deficiency, we need only replace that particular vitamin, and there is no upset in the balance of the other B vitamins.

Similarly, folic acid blood levels are sometimes reduced by the action of the drug sulphasalazine, used to treat ulcerative colitis. Taking aspirin for prolonged periods at high dose will reduce specifically the body vitamin C levels. Hence it would appear to be a sensible measure to supplement each of these drug treatments with the particular vitamin that is missing but this will not upset the balance of any of the other vitamins.

These are just a few examples where medicinal drugs affect the status of a specific vitamin in the body, but as we have seen there are many others. Once the vitamin deficiency is known it can be treated by simple supplementation to restore the body levels of that affected vitamin.

The best way to make the most of your fat-soluble vitamins is to remember that they are fats and that any factor upsetting fat absorption will have a deleterious effect upon the body status of the vitamins. Since they are fat-soluble, vitamins A, D, E and K will be retained in the body longer than water-soluble vitamins and will be stored in the liver and fatty tissues. It is because they are stored that, of all vitamins, A and D are regarded as the most toxic in high potency. Body levels can build up over a period of time until eventually a dangerous concentration is reached. By the same token, once this level is reached, even when they are no longer eaten, it takes a long time for the tissues to rid themselves of the excess vitamins. The safest way to get the most from vitamins A and D is not to go beyond the maximum daily intake recommended by the manufacturers. This is particularly so in the supplementation of babies and infants.

Any condition, drug or treatment such as liquid paraffin which can reduce the absorption of fats or can immobilise them will lead to deficiencies of the fat-soluble vitamins. If the interfering factor is long-lasting it could become essential to take these vitamins in some other way. One is by injection but a more feasible procedure for self-treatment is to take them as water-solubilized preparations. In this way the fat-absorption pathway is bypassed and the vitamins are treated as though they were water-soluble.

One of the biggest problems for those who wish to treat themselves with vitamins is how to get high levels of B12 into the body. This vitamin is unique because it requires attachment to a specific protein called intrinsic factor, which is produced in the parietal cells of the stomach, before it can be absorbed. The combination takes place in the stomach from whence the complex moves down to the part of the small intestine known as the ileum where in a specific area the whole complex is absorbed. The amount of vitamin B12 absorbed by this mechanism is unlikely to be above 8µg from a single dose since intrinsic factor production is limited and the receptor sites in the ileum soon become saturated.

However, in addition to this unique mechanism, some B12 is absorbed by simple diffusion. Radioactive tracer techniques carried out on pernicious anaemia patients, who have lost the ability to make intrinsic factor indicate that not more than 1 percent of a single dose of the vitamin is absorbed up to the 1,000µg level. Above this the percentage absorbed drops even further. What this means is that a normal individual taking 100µg of B12 in a single tablet will absorb only 9 (i.e. 1+8) µg. The rest is wasted. A person suffering from pernicious anaemia is unlikely to absorb more than one µg. There is a popular fallacy that sorbitol enhances the absorption of B12, even in pernicious anaemia patients, but the evidence for this is far from satisfactory.

We must, therefore, conclude that the only way in which to get high levels of B12 into the body is by intramuscular injection. Even by this route, probably 40 percent of a 1,000µg dose of cyanocobalamin is excreted in the first 24 hours but thereafter the excretion rate drops dramatically. The best type of vitamin B12 for intramuscular injection is hydroxocobalamin. Because this differs slightly in structure it is retained in the body to a much greater extent than cyanocobalamin. Pernicious anaemia patients who require regular injections of the vitamin usually respond satisfactorily to 1,000µg of hydroxo-cobalamin every two months, or to 1,000µg of cyanocobalamin monthly.

We have seen that once supplementation is decided upon we can, with a little thought, make the most of the many preparations that are available. The factors controlling our choice are to a large extent personal. Do we require an all-round multivitamin intake simply to insure against deficiency? Perhaps a rapid high-level intake is needed. Are we creating specific deficiencies by our way of life, whether they be due to lifestyle or medicinal drugs, and if so what are they? Let us make sure that we know exactly why we feel we need the vitamins we are taking. Once that is established, common sense will usually dictate how we may make the best use of them.

OTHER BOOKS FROM AMBERWOOD PUBLISHING ARE:

Aromatherapy Lexicon – The Essential Reference by Geoff Lyth and Sue Charles is a colourful, fun way to learn about Aromatherapy. £4.99.

Aromatherapy – The Baby Book by Marion Del Gaudio Mak. An easy to follow guide to massage for the infant or child. £3.99

Aromatherapy – Simply For You by Marion Del Gaudio Mak. A clear, simple and comprehensive guide to Aromatherapy for beginners. £2.99.

Aromatherapy – A Guide for Home Use by Christine Westwood. All you need to know about essential oils and using them. £1.99.

Aromatherapy – for Stress Management by Christine Westwood. Covering the use of essential oils for everyday stress-related problems. £3.50.

Aromatherapy – For Healthy Legs and Feet by Christine Westwood. A guide to the use of essential oils for the treatment of legs and feet. £2.99.

Aromatherapy – The Pregnancy Book by Jennie Supper RM RN MGCP. Jennie Supper, a State Registered Nurse and Midwife explains the use of Aromatherapy during pregnancy and the common conditions which may be treated safely. £5.99

Aromatherapy – A Nurses Guide by Ann Percival SRN. The ultimate, safe, lay guide to the natural benefits of Aromatherapy. Including recipes and massage techniques for many medical conditions and a quick reference chart. £2.99.

Aromatherapy – A Nurses Guide for Women by Ann Percival SRN. Concentrates on women's health for all ages. Including sections on PMT, menopause, infertility, cellulite. £2.99.

Aromatherapy – Essential Oils in Colour by Rosemary Caddy Bsc Hons, ARCS MISP is a unique book depicting the chemistry of essential oils. £9.99.

Aroma Science – The Chemistry & Bioactivity of Essential Oils by Dr Maria Lis-Balchin. With a comprehensive list of the Oils and scientific analysis. Includes sections on the sense of smell and the history of Aromatherapy. £5.99.

Woman Medicine – Vitex Agnus Castus by Simon Mills MA, FNIMH. The story of the herb that has been used for centuries in the treatment of women's problems. £2.99.

Plant Medicine – A Guide for Home Use (New Edition) by Charlotte Mitchell MNIMH. A guide to home use giving an insight into the wonderful healing qualities of plants. £2.99.

Ancient Medicine – Ginkgo Biloba (New Edition) by Dr Desmond Corrigan BSc(Pharms), MA, Phd, FLS, FPSI. Improved memory, circulation and concentration are associated with Ginkgo and explained in this book. £2.99.

Indian Medicine – The Immune System by Dr Desmond Corrigan BSc(Pharms), MA, Phd, FLS, FPSI. An intriguing account of the history of the plant called Echinacea and its power to influence the immune system. £2.99.

Herbal Medicine for Sleep & Relaxation by Dr Desmond Corrigan BSc(Pharms), MA, PhD, FLS, FPSI. A guide to the natural sedatives as an alternative to orthodox drug therapies, drawing on the latest medical research, presented in an easy reference format. £2.99.

Herbal First Aid by Andrew Chevallier BA, MNIMH. A beautifully clear reference book of natural remedies and general first aid in the home. £2.99.

Natural Taste – Herbal Teas, A Guide for Home Use by Andrew Chevallier BA, MNIMH. Contains a comprehensive compendium of Herbal Teas gives information on how to make it, its benefits, history and folklore. £3.50.

Garlic– How Garlic Protects Your Heart by Prof E. Ernst MD, PhD. Used as a medicine for over 4500 years, this book examines the latest scientific evidence supporting Garlic's effect in reducing cardiovascular disease, the Western World's number one killer. £3.99.

Phytotherapy – Fifty Vital Herbs by Andrew Chevallier, the most popular medicinal herbs with uses and advice written by an expert. £6.99

Insomnia – Doctor I Can't Sleep by Dr Adrian Williams FRCP. Written by one of the world's leading sleep experts, Dr Williams explains the phenomenon of sleep and sleeping disorders and gives advice on treatment. With 25% of the adult population reporting difficulties sleeping – this book will be essential reading for many. £2.99.

Eyecare Eyewear – For Better Vision by Mark Rossi Bsc, MBCO. A complete guide to eyecare and eyewear including an assessment of the types of spectacles and contact lenses available and the latest corrective surgical procedures. £3.99.

Arthritis and Rheumatism by Dr John Cosh FRCP, MD. Covers all forms of Arthritis, its effects and the treatments available. £4.95.

Feng Shui – A Guide for Home use by Karen Ward. Simple tips on "Power of Place" and effects of environment of health. £2.99